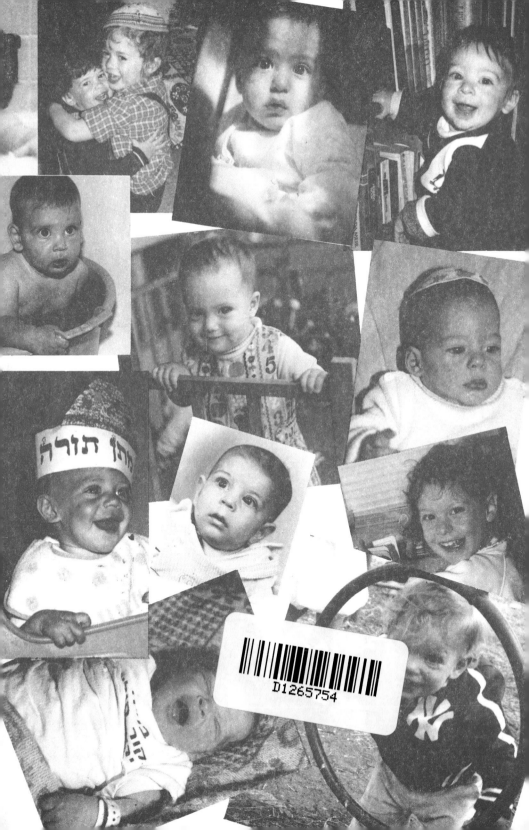

אדו תורה

D1265754

B'Sha'ah Tovah

RABBI BARUCH FINKELSTEIN

MICHAL FINKELSTEIN, R.N.

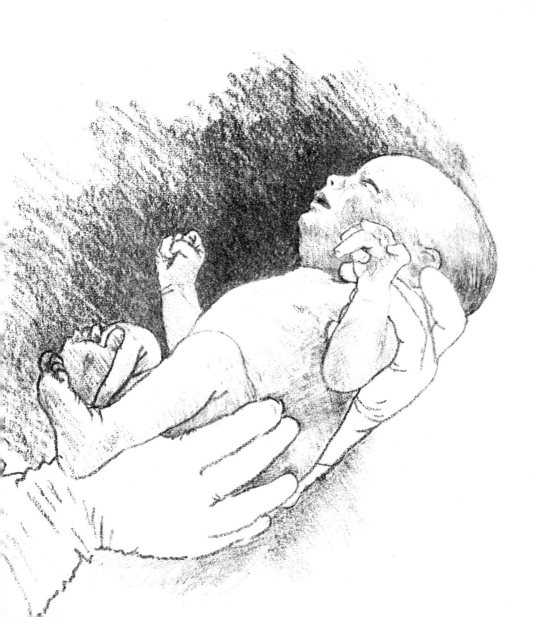

B'Sha'ah Tovah

The Jewish Woman's
Clinical and Halachic Guide
to Pregnancy and Childbirth

FELDHEIM PUBLISHERS Jerusalem / New York

Library of Congress Cataloging-in-Publication Data

Finkelstein, Baruch.
    B'sha'ah tovah : the Jewish woman's clinical & halachic guide
to pregnancy & childbirth / by Baruch Finkelstein and Michal
Finkelstein.
      p. cm.
    Includes index.
    ISBN 0-87306-629-4
    1. Pregnancy—Popular works. 2. Childbirth—Popular works.
3. Pregnancy—Religious aspects—Judaism. 4. Childbirth—
Religious aspects—Judaism. 5. Medical laws and legislation
(Jewish law) I. Finkelstein, Michal. II. Title. III. Title: B'sha'ah tovah.
RG525.F514 1993
618.2'4—dc20   93-9493

First published 1993

Edited by Marsi Tabak

FELDHEIM PUBLISHERS
200 Airport Executive Park
Nanuet, NY 10954

POB 35002
Jerusalem 91350

Printed in Israel

10   9   8   7   6   5   4

This book is dedicated by my lifelong friends,
Dave and Joan Hardoon, and Jonathan and Eden
Hardoon, to the memory of their beloved parents
and grandparents

Julius   *and*   **Cecil**

פנחס בן יוסף   זיסל בת בנימין

נפטר י״ז טבת תשל״א   נפטרה כ׳ אייר תשמ״ט

Seffer

Humble, always joyful, and an inspiration to us all.

תנצב״ה

In memory of my father

Sheldon Bank

שמעון הירש בן בנימין

נפטר נר ח׳ של חנוכה תשמ״ה

who returned his soul to his Maker
before he saw me become a mother

תנצב״ה

ב"ה, כ"ה כסלו תשנ"ג
18-2-93/נ"ג

הסכמה

"הלא כחלב תתיכני וכגבינה תקפיאני עור ובשר תלבישני ובעצמות וגידים
תשוככני חיים וחסד עשית עמדי ופקודתך שמרה רוחי" (איוב פרק י).

חז"ל הביאו זאת במסכת נדה דף כ"ה ע"א על יצירת הולד והקשו
התוס' וכן תוספות הרא"ש הרי כתוב ביחזקאל ל"ז "ונתתי עליכם גידים
והעלתי עליכם בשר וקרמתי עליכם עור ונתתי בכם רוח וחייתם וידעתם
כי אני ה'", משמע קודם גידים אח"כ בשר ואח"כ עור. ואילו באיוב
משמע קודם עור אח"כ בשר ואח"כ עצמות וגידין, ותירצו שבבריאת
הולד הסדר הוא עור ובשר תחילה ואח"כ עצמות וגידין. אולם בתחיית
המתים הסדר הפוך, בדומה לאדם שפושט וחוזר ולובש, שמה שפשט
אחרון לובש ראשון. זה נאמר על תחיית המתים. אך בתחילת בריאת
הולד עור ובשר תחילה ואח"כ עצמות וגידין.

התינוק שבמעי אמו הוא מפלאי הבריאה שבחסד הוא מתקיים —
"ופקודתך שמרה רוחי" — עפ"י הגמ' בברכות ס' ע"ב שאנחנו מברכים
"אשר יצר את האדם בחכמה וכו'" ומסיימים "מפליא לעשות" ופירש
רש"י ותוס' על הפסוק "כי גדול אתה ועושה נפלאות אתה אלקים לבדך"
אדם עושה נאד אפילו יש בו נקב אחד מלא מחט סידקית הרוח יוצא
ואינו יכול לשמור בו יין. והקב"ה ברא נקבים נקבים באדם ושומר הרוח
שאינו יוצא ממנו" תוס' שם והוסיף רש"י "וזוהי פליאה וחכמה".

וכן אומרת הגמ' בנדה ל' ע"ב "דרש רבי שמלאי למה הולד דומה במעי
אמו לפנקס שמקופל ומונח ידיו על שתי צדעיו... ופיו סתום וטבורו פתוח
ואוכל ממה שאמו אוכלת... וכיון שיצא לאויר העולם נפתח הסתום

ונסתם הפתוח שאילמלא כן אינו יכול לחיות אפילו שעה אחת... ואין לך
ימים שאדם שרוי בטובה יותר מאותן הימים (שנמצא במעי אמו) שנאמר
מי יתנני כירחי קדם כו'" וזה שאנחנו אומרים אשר יצר את האדם
בחכמה... שאם יפתח אחד מהם או יסתם אחד מהם א"א להתקיים
אפילו שעה אחת". הכוונה במעי אמו וכשיצא נפתח הסתום ונסתם
הפתוח שאם כן לא כן לא יכול להתקיים אפילו שעה אחת.

האבודרהם המובא בב"י סימן ו' הסביר שיי"מ רופא כל בשר ע"ש הנקבים
שברא בו להוציא פסולת מאכלו כי אם יתעפש בבטן ימות והוצאתו היא
רפואה וזהו רופא כל בשר ואומר ומפליא לעשות ע"ש שבורר בו הקב"ה
טוב המאכל ודוחה הפסולת ונכון הוא ע"כ. הוי אומר שיצירת האדם
וקיום האדם היא חכמה ופלא. ולפיכך כתוב בזוחה"ק פרשת שמות שמי
שגורם להפלה הוא סותר בניינו של הקב"ה וכן יש הלכות רבות כיצד על
האשה לנהוג בעת הריונה וכן הלכות רבות לפני ההריון.

יפה עשו איש ואשה שזכו ונהיו לקשר אחד והוציאו ספר מתוקן המיוסד
על מאמרי חז"ל הלכות הנחוצות בעניין הריון ולידה וגידול הילדים, וסתות
וטהרה וכו'. ה"ה משפ' הרב ברוך פינקלשטיין שליט"א, שמהשמים זיכו
להם להוציא ספר כזה מלוקט מראשונים ואחרונים, דברי הלכה ומוסר,
אגדה ומחשבה והכל נחצב מדברי חז"ל ודלו מים מבארותיו ואיישר
חילם שהפליאו לעשות בדבר זה.

יהי רצון שהקב"ה ימלא משאלות ליבכם לעבודתו יתברך ותתברכו בכל
מידי דמיטב, וכל אשר תפנו תשכילו ותצליחו ויהי ה' עמכם, אכי"ר.

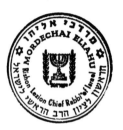

מרדכי אליהו
ראשון לציון הרב הראשי לישראל

Rabbi CHAIM P. SCHEINBERG
Rosh Hayeshiva "TORAH-ORE"
and Morah Hora'ah of Kiryat Mattersdorf

הרב חיים פינחס שיינברג
ראש ישיבת "תורה-אור"
ומורה הוראה דקרית מטרסדורף

בס"ד

שמח לבי בראותי לפני ספר שהוא מדריך לאשה היהודית על הריון ולידה אשר נכתב ע"י האי גברא יקירא הרב ר' ברוך פינקלשטיין שליט"א ונות ביתו מרת מיכל פינקלשטיין שתחי' מנב"ת.

זכו המחברים להניח על שולחן הלומדים ספר נחמד ומועיל העוסק בתהליך המופלאה של יצירת הולד ועל דרך היחודית שבה על שותפו של הקב"ה ביצירה להתבונן ולנהוג בכל אחד מהשלבים של גידולו.

דברי הרב המחבר מוגשים בבהירות ובטוב טעם ודעת ומבוססים על דעות גדולי ישראל מש"ס ומפוסקים מחכמי ספרד ואשכנז. ידיו רב לו ובכל ענין הוסיף ציונים למקור הדברים אשרי חילו לאורייתא. כ"כ דברי המחברת אשר שרתה שנים רבות כמילדת בביה"ח "ביקור חולים" בעיה"ק ירושלים יעילות ומרגיעות – מנוסחות היטיב, מלמדות ומדריכות את הקורא דרך יום וחודש משך כל תקופת ההריון. גם האיורים והטבלאות מובאות בצורה מהנה ובדרך שכל אחד בישראל יכול ללמוד מהם.

ואף כי אין בכוחי לשים עיני בכל עניני הספר, לכן אינני יכול לתת הסכמה על כל פרט ופרט, אבל ממליץ אני לכל משפחה להביא ברכה זו אל ביתו, ויזכו המחברים עוד רבות לזכות את הרבים להרבות משפחות בישראל אשר יהיו משכן להשכינה הקדושה ולדורות ישרים ומבורכים, ולהגדיל תורה ולהאדירה.

הכו"ח לכבוד התורה ולומדיה, פה עיה"ק ירושלים תובב"א.
ו' כסלו התשנ"ג

חיים פינחס שיינברג

רחוב פנים מאירות 2, ירושלים, ת. ד. 6979, טל. 371513־(02), ישראל
2, Panim Meirot St., Jerusalem, P. O. B. 6979, Tel (02)-371513, Israel

BIKUR CHOLIM HOSPITAL, JERUSALEM, ISRAEL

DEPARTMENT OF OBSTETRICS AND GYNECOLOGY

בית החולים בקור חולים ירושלים

מחלקת נשים ויולדות

12.1.93

חיבורם המשותף של הרב פינקלשטיין ואשתו המיילדת מיכל פינקלשטיין
מהווה סיכום יסודי ועניני בנושאים העוסקים באשה היהודיה, הריון,
לידה ומשכב הלידה.
החומר מוגש ברהיטות, מובא בצורה קריאה ביותר, קלה להבנה ועונה
על רוב רובם של השאלות המתעוררות בלב כל אשה המצפה ללידה.
עבודת הצוות בין הרב למיילדת נעשתה בצורה יסודית ועניינית כשהיא
קושרת בין תהליכים רפואיים והלכתיים ומאירה סוגיות רבות.
הקריאה קלה ומהנה ובטוחני שלימוד הספר יביא להורדת המתח שלקראת
סוף ההריון והלידה. הבנת התהליכים הקורים בזמן ההריון, הלידה
והשלב שלאחר מכן יכינו את האשה בצורה הטובה ביותר לקראת החוויה
הכבירה של הבאת יצור חי לעולם.

בכבוד רב,

ד"ר ח. יפה
מנהל מח' נשים ויולדות

This co-authored work by HaRav Baruch Finkelstein and his wife
Michal, a registered nurse and midwife, is a profound examination of
the topics of pregnancy, childbirth, and the postnatal period, in a
Jewish context.

The material is very readable, easy to understand and answers the
majority of questions that arise in the minds of pregnant women.

This joint effort of Rav and midwife combines the halachic and
clinical aspects and sheds light on a wide range of subjects.

The style of the book is light and enjoyable, and I am certain that
reading it will ease the tension and stress that often accompanies
pregnancy and childbirth. Understanding the processes that occur will
prepare the Jewish woman in the best way possible for the marvelous
experience of bringing new life into the world.

Dr. Chaim Yaffe
Head of the Gynecology and Obstetrics Dept.
Bikur Cholim Hospital, Jerusalem

5, STRAUSS ST. P.O.B. 492, JERUSALEM, 91004 ISRAEL, Tel. 701114-701261 ,701111 .טל ,91004 ,ירושלים ,492 .ת.ד ,5 שטראוס 'רח

Concerning the *Halachah* in this Book

1. Many times in this book the suggestion to "consult your Rav" appears, for one of the following reasons:

a. the *halachah* under discussion must always take into account the individual's personal situation;

b. there are differing opinions among contemporary *poskim* over the *halachah* under discussion;

c. the *halachah* under discussion may need further clarification; and/or

d. the custom observed by a particular family or community might be different from what is mentioned here.

2. The purpose of the footnotes is to credit a conclusive decision of a halachic authority but not to explain the origins and reasoning behind each *halachah.* For instance, if the *halachah* was decided by the *Magen Avraham* and cited in the *Mishnah Berurah,* the footnote will say "*Mishnah Berurah,*" usually with no mention of his source. However, it should be noted that certain *halachos* were explained either briefly or at length in the Hebrew appendix.

3. The transliterated footnotes are cited in order to inform the reader who is not yet fluent in Hebrew of the source of the *halachah.*

4. Only *halachos* that were thought to be most commonly needed are cited. Therefore, halachic situations dealing with, for example, *Yom Tov,* are not mentioned at all (with the exception of fast days).

5. Variations in Sephardic and Ashkenazic tradition have been taken into consideration.

6. Although this book contains halachic guidelines, it is always advisable and preferable to consult your Rav.

Concerning the Clinical Advice in this Book

The clinical advice in this book is intended to inform and educate, but is not intended to substitute for or fulfill your responsibility of consulting your physician. It is essential that you follow the advice of your physician and receive the treatments he/she deems necessary. Every case requires individualized medical attention and no book, regardless of its degree of professionalism or accuracy, can replace that.

ACKNOWLEDGMENTS

After over two years of a concerted writing effort, a great deal of *siyyata d'Shemaya*, and an accelerated finish, this work finally sees the light of day. As Yaakov Feldheim said to us at one point, "It's been a long pregnancy."

Due to the multifaceted content of this book, Michal and I sought out and benefited from the talents and expertise of many other professionals in various fields. It is therefore our pleasure to fulfill the words of *Chazal*: "One must acknowledge those from whom he benefited" (*Yalkut Torah* 133).

Our gratitude is extended to:

Ha-Rishon l'Tzion, Ha-Rav Ha-Gaon Mordechai Eliyahu, *shlita*, who supported the idea of this book from its inception and gave graciously of his precious time to discuss halachic matters;

Ha-Rav Ha-Gaon Chaim Pinchas Sheinberg, *shlita*, who discussed many of the *halachos* with me and offered sound advice on the correct approach in expressing them effectively;

Ha-Rav Ha-Gaon Zev Leff, *shlita*, for his inspiring and insightful Foreword. Rabbi Leff and his *Rabbanit* Rivkah have been close to us for many years, and we consider it a great honor that he could be a part of our project;

Dr. Chaim Yaffe, our medical consultant, who is head of Obstetrics and Gynecology at Jerusalem's Bikur Cholim Hospital. His genuine interest in this work was a tremendous source of encouragement, and he made himself constantly available to discuss the clinical aspects of the book;

Dr. Matityahu Erlichman, our pediatric consultant, who supplied us with research material and was always eager to advise us on various health issues;

my parents, Philip and Alice Finkelstein. Their continuous support was the catalyst for this undertaking;

my early childhood friend Jonathan Hardoon, whose generosity and unconditional friendship have never ceased, and his parents, Dave and Joan Hardoon, who since my youth have been like family to me. I am glad that they are a part of this project;

Leah Levenson and Monique Bebas, who taught Michal not only the professional aspects of midwifery, but the human aspects as well;

our good friend Mindy Ribner, the graphic artist whose skillful illustrations grace many of the pages here;

our fitness and exercise consultant, Leora Ashkenazi;

Mrs. Simchah Tabesky, an experienced childbirth educator, who reviewed selected sections of the book, and offered us her many constructive ideas;

my good friends Rabbi Chaim Block, *shlita,* and Dr. Chanoch Bronznick, who meticulously reviewed the halachic sections;

my good friend Ya'akov Snir of Jerusalem's Hebrew Studio, who translated the manuscript into Hebrew.

A very special thank you to my sister, Sheila Sodden, for her efficiency and swiftness in handling some very important last-minute details, which greatly enhanced the character of the book.

A special "*yasher ko'ach*" to Mr. Yaakov Feldheim and to his staff at Feldheim Publishers. Marsi Tabak, Feldheim's Editor-in-Chief, made this book "her baby" (pun intended). Mrs. Tabak's vision of what this book was supposed to be matched our own, and it was a pleasure to work with her and the Feldheim staff: Art Director Harvey Klineman; editors and proofreaders Bracha Steinberg, Rivka Mishmor, and Joyce Bennett; and typesetter Hannah Hartman. The entire staff was enthusiastic about the book, made valuable suggestions, and worked with dedication on every aspect of its production.

And last but certainly not least, we thank Rabbi Asher and Chana Margaliot, our initial editors, who prepared the manuscript for submission and whose literary proficiency was exceeded only by their enthusiasm for working on this project. They not only added commas and corrected spelling; they became an integral part of the work, and at times we felt as if they were our partners in writing this book. They were our first address to turn to when problems arose, or for consultation on style and content. We benefited greatly from their *chochmas chayim,* and consider it a *zechus* to have worked together with them as colleagues and very close friends.

May Hashem bless them all *ba-kol mi-kol kol.*

Although we thank Hashem every day in our *tefillos,* we would like to express our gratitude to Hashem for His many blessings: for giving Michal the *zechus* to be a part of so many people's *simchahs* in her professional capacity, which *Chazal* have called "*chochmah*"; for giving me the greatest *zechus* of all — to sit *b'ohalah shel Torah;* and for giving us the wonderful opportunity to live in Eretz Yisrael and raise our family here. May we soon be joined by all of *Am Yisrael.*

Throughout the writing of this book, we felt we had been given a special *shelichus.* We humbly pray that Hashem will bless our endeavor, that it may benefit Jewish families everywhere.

Baruch and Michal Finkelstein
Rosh Chodesh Nissan 5753

Contents

by Rabbi Zev Leff
Rav of Moshav Matityahu

The portion of the Torah which deals with childbirth and its pertinent laws is curiously sandwiched between the laws concerning kosher and non-kosher varieties of animals, birds and fish, and the laws of *tzara'as*, the quasi-physical ailment visited upon those who engage in gossip and slander. From this juxtaposition we may infer the true significance of childbirth.

Turnus Rufus, the wicked Roman general, once challenged Rabbi Akiva: "Which is superior — that which God makes, or that which man makes?" He expected Rabbi Akiva to reply that God's handiwork is certainly superior. Then he would have countered that the uncircumcised non-Jew who remains as God made him is superior to the circumcised Jew. However, Rabbi Akiva unexpectedly replied that most certainly that which man makes is superior.

Turnus Rufus, caught off guard, questioned the truth of this contention, and Rabbi Akiva answered with his own question: When he returned home for his meal, would Turnus Rufus prefer to eat the simpler kernels of wheat that God produced or the refined bread and cake made by his wife? Obviously, the bread and cake are superior to the wheat. Rabbi Akiva wished to demonstrate that God created an imperfect world where He provided only the raw materials, intending that man should perfect the world, and himself along with it, both physically and spiritually.

In this respect, man is God's partner in Creation, picking up where God left off, as it were. In fact, some commentaries interpret the words of the Torah, *"Asher bara Elokim la'asos,"* as "the world which God created for man to develop."

The Talmud comments on the verse "*Adam l'amal yul-lad* — Man is born to toil" (*Iyov* 5:7) — that every human being was created to develop himself and the world around him, ever striving towards perfection. This toil, although most certainly including the improvement of the material world through physical effort, is expressed most intensely in man's ability to speak and communicate. It is this toil of the mouth which uniquely characterizes the human being and sets him apart from the animal world.

Although this verbal toil consists of communication, its most exalted form is Torah study. Man's mission in this world is an ongoing quest to know his Creator and to strive to emulate Him. This recognition is in reality part of man's innate being. The Rabbis relate that throughout the nine months of development within the womb, the fetus is taught the entire Torah by an angel. Upon birth, the angel strikes the child on the mouth and causes him to forget everything that he has learned. It seems strange that God would ordain such an exercise in futility — nine months of learning doomed to be completely forgotten! In addition, the manner in which this knowledge is eliminated needs explanation. Why is the target the mouth and not the brain? After all, memory is located in the brain and not in the mouth.

In the *alef-beis* there are two variations of the letter *peh*: *peh pasu'ach*, literally the open *peh* at the end of the word; and *peh sasum*, the closed *peh* at the beginning and the middle of the word. The letter *peh* represents the mouth, which has two functions: the closed mouth that ingests and chews the food to prepare it for integration into the body by the digestive system (one chews with his mouth closed, hence the beginning of the digestive process begins when the mouth closes on the food that has been put into it); and the open mouth that conveys speech.

Man enhances and realizes his potential as a partner

in Creation by maintaining and expanding his physical being through eating, and by expressing his spiritual essence verbally through Torah learning, prayer, and communication with others. In this view, the tongue is referred to as *lashon*, related to the word *lash*, which means to prepare and knead dough. Just as in the process of kneading dough a liquid and solid are combined to create the dough, so, too, the tongue takes the ideas and concepts that compose the inner spiritual essence of man and encloses them in a verbal framework which gives them expression in the material world.

The womb is the place where the foundation of man's ultimate potential is developed. His physical essence is provided jointly by his father and mother and is nurtured by the mother's body. His spiritual essence, on the other hand, is supplied by God and nurtured by His angel, who implants a recognition of the totality of spirituality, a knowledge of his Creator which is the essence of Torah.

During this time the child's mouth has no function in the nourishment process. It is as if it is tightly shut. The baby is passive — doing nothing to develop or enhance his own existence. At birth, man begins to take action. Although he is still dependent on his mother to provide his sustenance, he uses his mouth to actively participate in ingesting the food which will enhance his physical being. Similarly, although he is still dependent on his parents to develop his ability to learn and express himself, he opens his mouth to actively express himself verbally.

Therefore the angel strikes the child on the mouth, marking the transition between the initial stages of his life. In the womb the fetus was totally passive, as if with a closed mouth, unable to utilize that mouth to fulfill his mission of perfecting himself and the world around him physically and spiritually. Once he is born, however, his mouth opens to begin the toil that is his *raison d'être* in this world.

Thus man is gradually prepared for the self-perfection

he must actively achieve in this world as a partner in the ongoing process of Creation. He begins by passively receiving his potential and continues with a period of education and training lasting twelve years for a girl and thirteen years for a boy. During this time, the parents direct and share in this quest for perfection, paving the way for the child until he is able to take the reins and become a fully responsible and accountable free agent, who can actively choose to be a partner in God's plan for ultimate world perfection.

This is the spirit of the blessing a father makes at his son's bar mitzvah: "*Baruch she'petarani mi-onsho shel zeh* — Blessed is God Who has exempted me from being responsible for this child." This blessing reflects the joy of seeing one's child capable of accepting the responsibility for his own actions — accountable, functional, and thus able to realize and fulfill his sacred mission in life. From this standpoint, the same blessing applies equally to a girl at bas mitzvah, but is not actually recited because of other considerations.

As man realizes his potential and enhances his being physically and spiritually by recognizing his Creator, emulating Him and conveying this to others, he becomes aware that he has a responsibility to transmit and perpetuate this recognition beyond his own mortal lifetime. He therefore becomes a partner in Creation in an immortal, eternal manner — through the act of procreation. When the parent transmits to his child the spiritual values and truths he has learned and embodied, the child also becomes the spiritual continuation of the parent. In this vein, *Chazal* relate, he who is survived by righteous children is considered as one who did not die. Thus the child is the physical continuation of the parent.

It is now apparent why the *parashah* of birth is sandwiched between kosher animals and the laws of *tzara'as.* Man must promote his physical existence by eating kosher food, and enhance his spiritual development by utilizing his tongue in kosher speech. For this reason, the sections which deal with the dual function of the mouth, which represents man's quest for personal growth and perfection, circumscribe the phenomenon of birth, which represents the perpetuation of that quest, thus conferring upon it reason and purpose.

The first man and woman dealt capriciously with the immortal life they were given, not appreciating its full value and meaning. After their sin, God ordained that life would not come easily to man. He would have to endure difficulties and travail to secure the physical wherewithal to provide his livelihood. This travail was not a punishment, but rather a corrective measure to force man to contemplate his life and its true importance, as one tends to take things for granted when they come effortlessly and without difficulties.

Difficulties and problems force man to consider, reflect, ponder, deliberate, and ultimately to appreciate what he achieves. Similarly, man's spiritual quest is not effortless and painless, for here, too, he must labor to achieve spiritual perfection. In immortalizing his quest for perfection physically and spiritually by becoming God's partner in procreation, man must undergo pain and difficulty. Raising children is also no easy task, but is fraught with trials and tribulations, all for the purpose of inducing one to contemplate the value of the precious task with which he has been entrusted.

In this light, my dear long-time friends, Rabbi Baruch and Mrs. Michal Finkelstein, have done a great service to the Torah community by co-authoring this phenomenal book, B'Sha'ah Tovah: The Jewish Woman's Complete Clinical and Halachic Guide to Pregnancy and Childbirth, which deals with both the physical and spiritual aspects of bringing children into the world. They have provided a true Torah framework in which to better ponder and appreciate the miracle of birth.

May Hashem bless them for supplying the community with this valuable aid, and may they merit seeing the nachas of their effort crowned with success, and experiencing personal *Yiddishe nachas* from their children and children's children forever.

May we all strive to fulfill our purpose in this world, toiling endlessly towards perfection, towards the day when "God will give all nations a clear language to call upon His Name and serve Him shoulder to shoulder," and the entire world "will be filled with the knowledge of Hashem, as the waters cover the sea," soon in our days.

INTRODUCTION

In response to the need for spiritual growth in today's modern, sophisticated society, Jewish women are learning more Torah than in years past. An abundance of Torah publications, covering a wide range of topics — *halachah, mussar*, Bible commentary, Jewish thought, biographies of *tzaddikim*, and even religious works of fiction — are rapidly filling up our bookshelves. And yet, pregnancy and childbirth, the subject that seems to be a most dominant factor in our lives, has until now not found a place among our Jewish literature.

A woman's interest in childrearing begins in her toddler years. We have seen this with our daughters, whose favorite pastime, from the time they are old enough to walk, is pushing their dollies in baby carriages, dressing them, feeding them and pretending to be "Imma." Their imagination reflects an instinctive affinity for motherhood. This same natural interest is expressed when we women get together with our friends, for it seems that *our* favorite pastime is talking about pregnancy, childbirth and childrearing. Though our careers, hobbies and intellectual pursuits are also important to us, nothing fulfills us more than our accomplishments as mothers.

Preparation for motherhood begins with preparation for childbirth. It has been proven that proper preparation can make the difference between a positive birth experience and one that is negative and unpleasant. Ignorance is *not* bliss! Lack of knowledge can breed fear, anxiety and mistrust, which can transform the childbearing adventure into a frightening event and even cause unnecessary complications in delivery.

When the expectant mother understands and is more sensitive to the changes that are occurring in her body, she feels more in control and secure. The educated patient is able to communicate better with the medical staff, thus improving the quality of the care she receives. Whether giving birth for the first or the ninth time, there is always something to learn and prepare for, as each birth is different and special.

A Jewish woman has a unique lifestyle, and is interested in more than just the clinical aspects of childbirth. First and foremost, she needs to know how pregnancy and childbirth are viewed from a Torah perspective, to understand their significance. And, of course, she must be aware of the pertinent *halachos*: She is concerned with knowing not only how many contractions indicate true labor, but also how they will affect her status in terms of the Laws of Family Purity; she is concerned with knowing not only which prenatal tests are "safe," but which are halachically permissible and under what circumstances.

We who are so proud of our roles as mothers and look forward to having many children, need a pregnancy and childbirth book that speaks to us.

B'sha'ah Tovah clearly addresses the specific needs of the Jewish woman. This book is more than a combination of clinical information and *halachah*; it is a blend of the *kodesh* and *chol* — the sacred and the mundane — that reveals this topic as an entirely Jewish experience. With the publication of *B'sha'ah Tovah*, we are no longer limited to other clinical texts which express and illustrate ideas that are foreign or even contradictory to our Jewish way of life. *B'sha'ah Tovah* is the one childbirth book that can be introduced without reservations into every Jewish home and read by every mother- and father-to-be.

My experience as a midwife and public-health nurse has prepared me to present a complete clinical survey of pregnancy and childbirth which is based on the most current research and literature in the field. This is complemented by my husband's research into the wisdom of *Chazal* regarding health guidelines, physiology and pregnancy. My husband compiled the halachic information, and supplied inspirational Torah thoughts corresponding with each phase of childbearing and motherhood. Together, with Hashem's help, we have attempted to provide practical, pertinent and up-to-date information, to make this text a valuable reference guide.

B'Sha'ah Tovah will, God willing, occupy a prominent place in every Jewish woman's library. It will teach you, guide you and inspire you.

I hope you enjoy it.

Michal Finkelstein

...She is your companion, and wife of your covenant. (MALACHI 2:14)

The ideal union of husband and wife is an almost literal interpretation of the phrase "*Ishto k'gufo* — His wife is like his [own] body," as it is written in *Bereshis* 2:24: "And he shall cleave unto his wife and they shall be one flesh." The saintly Reb Aryeh Levin, *zt"l*, demonstrated the actualization of this notion when he brought his ailing wife to the doctor and said, "Her leg hurts us."

At the moment of childbirth the spiritual bond between husband and wife reaches its pinnacle, for it is the supreme expression of their *binyan adei ad* — their "edifice of eternity." The merit and burden of childbirth are the wife's, yet every husband feels he is an integral part of the childbearing experience as well. Many husbands, however, feel inadequately prepared to be of significant benefit to their wives during labor and delivery. Whether the expectant father is pacing the hospital corridors or sitting by the bedside attempting to comfort her, he is plagued by a sense of helplessness at his wife's most critical hour. He wishes he could do more.

The prenatal and post-partum stages of pregnancy require support as well. Before and after childbirth, hormonal changes can bring on mood swings in a woman. The anxieties of childbirth and motherhood, along with a possible feeling of discomfort due to weight gain, physical changes, and various aches and pains, may have strong influences on her emotional state.

Whether it is in the prenatal, perinatal or post-partum stage, the support that you can offer is not so much in the physical sphere but in the psychological and emotional. By showing concern and understanding, you can enable your wife to feel that pregnancy and childbirth

are a process that you are going through together. This will
alleviate much of the emotional stress that she may have
and boost her self-confidence. By being assured that you
— the most important person in her life — are beside her,
she can view childbirth as an exciting experience for both
of you.

In order to show understanding, a husband must be
knowledgeable. How can you reassure your wife if you
are even more nervous and unsure than she is? It is
therefore most beneficial for you to acquaint yourself
with at least some of the basic aspects of pregnancy and
childbirth.

Although this book is addressed primarily to the expectant mother, the expectant father who wishes to be
more aware and more involved will gain enormously
from reading it as well. *B'Sha'ah Tovah* was written in a
Torah spirit that will allow every Jewish husband the opportunity to educate himself in this area, and thereby
strengthen the bond between him and his wife at this
very sensitive and joyful time.

Most importantly, a thorough understanding of the
birth process will increase a couple's appreciation of
Hashem *Yisbarach.* In *Yesodei Ha-Torah,* the Rambam
writes that contemplating the ways and wondrous creations of Hashem brings one to love and fear God and
causes one to be overcome with a burning desire to
know his Creator. A profound appreciation can be obtained when you realize that a wondrous creation is happening right in your own home. During the development
and birth of your son or daughter, the greatness and
kindness of Hashem can be seen ever so clearly, and so
close at hand. You will feel impelled to reflect on your
own creation and birth as well, and fulfill the words of
David *Ha-Melech:* "I acknowledge You, for I am
awesomely, wondrously fashioned; wondrous are Your
works and my soul knows it well" (*Tehillim* 139:14; *see*
Radak).

It is our heartfelt prayer that your child be born with

Hakadosh Baruch Hu's goodness, blessing, grace and compassion. May he or she become a source of pride and joy for you and your wife, and may the birth take place *b'sha'ah tovah u'mutzlachas.*

Baruch Finkelstein

PART ONE:

The Prenatal Phase

1 | The Jewish Woman

The wisdom of women builds her home.
MISHLEI 14:1

A GREAT POWER FOR LIFE

On February 7, 1942, the Nazis issued a devastating decree against the Jewish ghetto of Kovno. They outlawed pregnancy for Jewish women. The penalty for a Jewish woman having a baby was her summary execution together with her newborn child.

Imagine the anguish of the pregnant women who realized that under Nazi occupation labor pains would signal not the beginning of life, but rather the end of life. Nevertheless, the Jewish women decided that instead of aborting their unborn children, they would have their babies and try to hide them from the Nazis.

Reb Itzchok Bloch was married for five years without being blessed with children, but shortly after the Nazi decree, his wife became pregnant. They searched out the safest hiding place and decided on the basement of the city's vocational school. Since it was located on the main road, they hoped that the traffic noise would muffle their baby's cries.

When they were blessed with a son, they arranged to make his *bris milah* in their makeshift home. The very moment that the *mohel* took the knife in his hand, a car

pulled up to the entrance of the school and Gestapo offi-
cers stepped out. The *mohel*'s hands trembled. The ema-
ciated faces of the small group gathered to celebrate this
auspicious occasion seemed to beg for a solution to their
dilemma. How could they save mother and baby from
the firing squad?

Finally, the silence was broken. The mother cried out,
"Hurry! Hurry! Circumcise the baby *now* — at least he
can die as a Jew!" The baby was circumcised, miraculously undetected by the Gestapo.[1]

The phenomenon of Jewish women risking their lives
in order to bear children is not unique to the hunger-
stricken ghetto of Kovno. Nor is it just another expression of heroic resistance to oppression. Rather it is the
manifestation of the essence of the Jewish woman and
the foundation upon which the entire Jewish nation is
built.

When the Jews were slaves to Pharaoh in Egypt, he
ordered the Jewish midwives to kill every Jewish male
child [in utero].[2] The midwives not only defied his cruel
decree, but even took special care of the babies after delivery.[3] When asked how they dared to disobey the order
of the mighty Pharaoh, they replied simply that "Hebrew
women are not like the Egyptian women, for they are
chayos — lively." The Ibn Ezra defines this as Jewish
women having a great power for life.[4]

Seeing that he could not succeed in corrupting the
midwives, Pharaoh decided to take matters into his own
hands. He ordered that all Jewish newborn males be
thrown into the Nile. When Amram, the leader of the
People, heard Pharaoh's new decree, he lost all hope.
How could he endure the horror of seeing the fruits of
his marital relationship drowned? In his despair, he preferred to divorce his wife, and all the other men soon followed his example.

Amram's daughter Miriam admonished her father,
saying, "Your decree is worse than Pharaoh's. His decree
eliminates only the male children, but your decision af-

fects the female ones as well. His decree pertains only to
this world, while your decision holds sway both in this
world and the next. It is questionable whether or not
Pharaoh's decree will be successful, but yours will surely
succeed." Thus Miriam convinced Amram to remarry his
wife Yocheved, and the other men also followed suit and
remarried their wives.[5]

THE SACRED MIRRORS

Even after the marriages were reestablished, the Jewish
men, drained by back-breaking labor, had little desire to
be with their wives. In addition, they were psychologically depressed by the life of hopeless suffering and suppression. They saw no reason to bring children into a
world of slavery, a common response among those living
under severe oppression.

Their wives, on the other hand, did not give up hope.
They believed in a better future. No matter how hard
their lives were at present, they still desired to build a
family. They realized that only by fulfilling the commandment to be fruitful and multiply could they
strengthen the Jewish People. Therefore, they enticed
their husbands, using shiny copper mirrors to beautify
themselves, and they succeeded in becoming pregnant.

Years later, when Hashem redeemed the Jews from
Egyptian bondage, and the women donated these same
shiny copper mirrors to the *Mishkan,* Moshe *Rabbenu*
misunderstood the significance of the mirrors and
deemed their use in the *Mishkan* improper. He said,
"How can I accept them? They are tools of the *yetzer ha-
ra.*" But Hashem told him to accept the mirrors, saying
"Do not despise these mirrors. It is because of them that
Bnei Yisrael multiplied in Egypt. The Jewish women
used them for the sake of Heaven, to beautify themselves
in order to continue bearing children despite the Egyptian torture, and therefore they are more precious to Me
than any other donation."

The mirrors, which the women used to prepare them-

selves for their husbands, were melted down to make the
kiyor, the wash basin where the *kohanim* prepared
themselves for the Divine Service.[6] The message is clear:
A woman who adorns herself for her husband's sake
with the holy intention of building a family is as sacred
as the *kohanim* preparing themselves for the Divine
Service.

KIYUM HA-OLAM

Hashem yearns for constant growth and development in
the world. He therefore established within nature the
ability to procreate. Every living thing — from a single
cell to plants and animals — reproduces.

Hashem blessed us to be fruitful and to multiply.[7]
With this commandment Hashem instilled in man the
physiological and psychological need to reproduce. Our
Sages tell us that the basis for man's determination to
advance, achieve, create, compete, explore, and rule is
rooted in the physiological need to be fruitful and multiply and fill the land.[8]

In woman this force is much stronger. It is not merely
the source of our determination. It is our very essence.
This "great power for life" gives us the strength to bear
the pains of labor. It gives us the hope to bring a new
generation into the world, even when bound by the
shackles of Egypt. It gives us the courage to bear children and circumcise them, even under threat of the Nazi
guillotine in Kovno.

Our innate desire to give life is even greater than the
instinct for self-preservation. That is why Pharaoh could
not compel the Jewish midwives to obey his decree. For
Hashem blessed Jewish women with a force that Pharaoh could never envisage — "a great power for life."

Therefore *Hakadosh Baruch Hu* bestowed upon
woman the responsibility to bear children and raise
them properly, thus fulfilling His principal desire: *kiyum
ha-olam* — the maintenance of the universe. To this end,
He fashioned our bodies with the unique suitability to

sustain and care for a baby: wide hips to accommodate the baby's birth, and breasts to nurse. He also gave woman a greater measure of the necessary character traits — understanding, sympathy, and patience — to nurture children and educate them to good *middos*.

According to *Chazal*, a man's body is comprised of 248 parts, while a woman's body has 252 parts.[9] The additional organs in the woman's body are for reproduction. Interestingly, the sum of 248 and 252 is 500, the same numerical value as the total of the letters in the words of "*P'ru u'revu* — Be fruitful and multiply."[10]

In the next few chapters, we will explore the scientific processes of reproduction, from conception through birth, which are, in effect, the development and fulfillment of *kiyum ha-olam* as Hashem intended.

NOTES

1. *Ani Ma'amin* (Jerusalem: Mossad Harav Kook), p. 93.
2. *Shemos* 1:16; see *Torah Temimah.*
3. Rashi, *Shemos* 1:17.
4. *Shemos* 1:19; see Ibn Ezra, "*Ki chayos hennah.*"
5. *Sotah* 12a.
6. *See* Rashi, *Shemos* 38:8.
7. *See* Rashi and Ramban, *Bereshis* 9:7.
8. *See Bereshis Rabbah* 9:7, "For without the *yetzer ha-ra*, a man would not build a house, marry, have children, or do business."
9. *Bechoros* 45a.
10. M. Glazerson, *Revelations about Marriage* (Jerusalem: Raz Ot Institute), p. 94.

2 | Fertilization

> There are three partners in man: the Holy
> One Blessed Be He, his father and his mother.
> NIDDAH 31a

**The Female
Reproductive
System**

Any discussion of the fertilization process must begin with the OVA (eggs). They are bred in the OVA-
RIES, which are small almond-shaped organs
located on each side of the uterus. Already in the
fetal stage, the ovaries contain several million oocytes
(immature ova) located in follicle cells. These follicle cells
are like egg crates safeguarding the eggs.

Despite the enormous quantity of eggs which are potentially available, by the time a girl reaches puberty,
normal degeneration has cut the number to about
400,000. From the onset of puberty, hormones influence
some of these follicles to grow and develop, resulting in
the release of one ovum each month. This is called OVU-
LATION. Over the 30-40 reproductive years, only about
400 out of the 400,000 follicles mature into eggs and are
released from the ovary.[1]

On the average, a girl begins to menstruate at the age
of twelve.[2] During the menstrual years, hormonal
changes occur on a daily, weekly and monthly basis.
These changes are controlled by messages relayed back
and forth between the hypothalamus and the pituitary
gland in the brain. The hypothalamus is the master con-

troller which transmits a "releasing factor" to the anterior (front) portion of the pituitary gland. The pituitary then acts to produce hormones which stimulate the ovaries to initiate and influence the menstrual cycle. The menstrual cycle is about 26 to 30 days in most women. Ovulation occurs midway through the menstrual cycle.

Once the egg is released from the ovary, it travels through the FALLOPIAN TUBES on its way to the uterus. It is in these smooth and narrow tubes that fertilization may occur. If fertilization does not take place, the unfertilized egg will dissolve, and the uterine lining (ENDOMETRIUM) which developed to receive the fertilized egg will fall away at the end of the cycle, causing the bleeding, which we call a period.

The UTERUS is a hollow, muscular, pear-shaped organ located between the bladder and the rectum in the pelvis. A few days after the ovum has been fertilized in the fallopian tube, it will implant itself in the uterus. From that moment a rapid and phenomenal growth process begins. The fertilized ovum develops into a complete human being while the uterus expands around it to nurture and protect it.

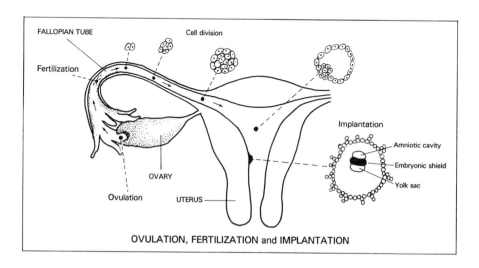

OVULATION, FERTILIZATION and IMPLANTATION

At the end of the pregnancy, the developed muscula-
ture of the uterus is even responsible for expelling the
baby. The uterus weighs only 2 oz. (60 gr.) at the beginning of the pregnancy, but will expand to 32 oz. (900
gr.). Likewise it starts at the length of 2 in. (5 cm.), and
eventually stretches until it reaches from the pelvic cav-
ity to the breastbone.

The Hebrew word for the uterus is *rechem*, from the
word *lerachem/rachamim*, meaning mercy. The function
of the uterus epitomizes the term mercy, for it takes care
of all of the baby's needs.

The Fertilization Process   Fertilization begins with the union of the sperm
and the egg. Although millions of sperm cells are
released, Rashi tells us that only the strongest and
best reach the ovum.[3] Sperm encounter many ob-
stacles on the journey toward their goal. In fact, most
sperm are destroyed by the acidic fluids normally found
in the birth canal. At the time of ovulation, however, cervical secretions are less viscous, more watery and more
alkaline, facilitating the transport and survival of sperm.
Although many sperm never reach their final destination, those that are successful reach the cervix in only
90 seconds, and only five minutes later arrive in the fallopian tubes, the site of fertilization.[4]

Only one sperm cell (spermatozoon) can penetrate the
wall of the ovum and fertilize it. Immediately after the
spermatozoon enters the ovum, a protective membrane
forms to prevent any other sperm from entering the
ovum. When an ovum is fertilized by a spermatozoon of
poor quality, the fertilized ovum is usually aborted in the
menstrual flow, without the mother ever being aware
that fertilization had occurred.[5]

Proper timing is essential to achieve fertilization.
Marital relations must take place within 24 hours of
ovulation, as the life span of the ovum is only 24 hours,
and sperm live up to 48 hours.

Each sperm and ovum carry 23 chromosomes which
combine to create a total of 46 chromosomes after fer-

tilization. Chromosomes are the cell components which transmit hereditary factors. Two of these 46 chromosomes determine the sex of the newborn. The ovum always transmits an X (female) chromosome, and the sperm can transmit either an X or a Y (male) chromosome. If an X-carrying spermatozoon fertilizes the ovum, the child will be a girl, and if a Y-carrying spermatozoon penetrates, the child will be a boy.

Detection of Pregnancy

The earliest and most common symptoms of pregnancy are fatigue, dizziness, and often nausea. When these symptoms are present and coincide with a missed period, it is usually merely a formality to have a pregnancy test confirm the suspected pregnancy.

Three to four days after conception, the fertilized ovum implants itself in the wall of the uterus and begins to secrete the hormone, human chorionic gonadotropin (hCG), into the mother's blood. A blood test called the beta-subunit assay can detect pregnancy as early as nine days after conception.

A urinalysis to detect pregnancy, urinary hCG, may be used more often as it is less expensive than the Beta hCG blood test. The hCG in the urine can be accurately detected 1-2 days after a missed period.

At-home pregnancy urinalysis is also inexpensive and offers 99% accuracy.

Ectopic Pregnancy

A fertilized ovum which implants itself anywhere other than in the uterus is termed an ectopic pregnancy. Although the majority of ectopic pregnancies occur in the fallopian tubes, implantation can also occur on the ovaries, intestines or cervix. The usual course of an ectopic pregnancy is that it grows until it bursts through the fallopian tube. Therefore, if a woman experiences a sharp, stabbing pain in one of the lower abdominal quadrants, accompanied by light to heavy bleeding, she should immediately seek medical attention. Other symptoms to watch out for are light-headedness and rapid pulse caused by internal bleeding. Ectopic pregnancy is usually treated by surgery to repair or remove the ruptured fallopian tube. Most women conceive again and have normal pregnancies.

Calculating the Due Date   Before discussing monthly fetal growth and development, it is helpful to understand how the date of conception and date of delivery are calculated. The clinical view of gestational age is almost always expressed in terms of weeks, not months. Of course, no woman functions like a textbook, and there is a wide range of days when a woman may ovulate or menstruate. Since the exact time of fertilization is not known, doctors simply calculate the gestational age and the due date from the first day of the last menstrual period, counting 280 days or 40 weeks.

The woman who knows when she went to the *mikveh* may estimate a different gestational date or due date from the one her doctor calculated. Any significant discrepancies between possible due dates should be discussed with the doctor.

Ultrasonic examinations can accurately measure a fetus' head and femur (thighbone) size, thereby estimating its gestational age. See Chapter 4 on Prenatal Care for a more thorough discussion of ultrasound.

The Gemara predicts delivery 271 days after conception.[6] Even the *gematria* of the Hebrew word for pregnancy — *herayon* — is 271. In Talmudic times, women's cycles were very precise. Today, however, the cycles are less exact — so much so that forty percent of women do not even deliver within a seven-day radius of their estimated due date.[7]

Jewish significance can also be attributed to the modern calculation of 280 days from the menstrual cycle. The number forty symbolizes preparation: forty years of wandering through the desert before entering *Eretz Yisrael*; forty days before birth a person's spouse is designated for him in Heaven;[8] and a person must have forty years of learning before being considered qualified to render halachic decisions.[9] The number seven symboli-

To determine your due date, find the date of the first day of your last period in the rows of small type. The date in bold immediately below it (280 days later) is your projected due date.

	1	2	3	4	5	6	7	8	9	10	11	12	13	14	15	16	17	18	19	20	21	22	23	24	25	26	27	28	29	30	31	
JANUARY	1	2	3	4	5	6	7	8	9	10	11	12	13	14	15	16	17	18	19	20	21	22	23	24	25	26	27	28	29	30	31	JANUARY
OCTOBER	8	9	10	11	12	13	14	15	16	17	18	19	20	21	22	23	24	25	26	27	28	29	30	31	1	2	3	4	5	6	7	NOVEMBER
FEBRUARY	1	2	3	4	5	6	7	8	9	10	11	12	13	14	15	16	17	18	19	20	21	22	23	24	25	26	27	28				FEBRUARY
NOVEMBER	8	9	10	11	12	13	14	15	16	17	18	19	20	21	22	23	24	25	26	27	28	29	30	1	2	3	4	5				DECEMBER
MARCH	1	2	3	4	5	6	7	8	9	10	11	12	13	14	15	16	17	18	19	20	21	22	23	24	25	26	27	28	29	30	31	MARCH
DECEMBER	6	7	8	9	10	11	12	13	14	15	16	17	18	19	20	21	22	23	24	25	26	27	28	29	30	31	1	2	3	4	5	JANUARY
APRIL	1	2	3	4	5	6	7	8	9	10	11	12	13	14	15	16	17	18	19	20	21	22	23	24	25	26	27	28	29	30		APRIL
JANUARY	6	7	8	9	10	11	12	13	14	15	16	17	18	19	20	21	22	23	24	25	26	27	28	29	30	31	1	2	3	4		FEBRUARY
MAY	1	2	3	4	5	6	7	8	9	10	11	12	13	14	15	16	17	18	19	20	21	22	23	24	25	26	27	28	29	30	31	MAY
FEBRUARY	5	6	7	8	9	10	11	12	13	14	15	16	17	18	19	20	21	22	23	24	25	26	27	28	1	2	3	4	5	6	7	MARCH
JUNE	1	2	3	4	5	6	7	8	9	10	11	12	13	14	15	16	17	18	19	20	21	22	23	24	25	26	27	28	29	30		JUNE
MARCH	8	9	10	11	12	13	14	15	16	17	18	19	20	21	22	23	24	25	26	27	28	29	30	31	1	2	3	4	5	6		APRIL
JULY	1	2	3	4	5	6	7	8	9	10	11	12	13	14	15	16	17	18	19	20	21	22	23	24	25	26	27	28	29	30	31	JULY
APRIL	7	8	9	10	11	12	13	14	15	16	17	18	19	20	21	22	23	24	25	26	27	28	29	30	1	2	3	4	5	6	7	MAY
AUGUST	1	2	3	4	5	6	7	8	9	10	11	12	13	14	15	16	17	18	19	20	21	22	23	24	25	26	27	28	29	30	31	AUGUST
MAY	8	9	10	11	12	13	14	15	16	17	18	19	20	21	22	23	24	25	26	27	28	29	30	31	1	2	3	4	5	6	7	JUNE
SEPTEMBER	1	2	3	4	5	6	7	8	9	10	11	12	13	14	15	16	17	18	19	20	21	22	23	24	25	26	27	28	29	30		SEPTEMBER
JUNE	8	9	10	11	12	13	14	15	16	17	18	19	20	21	22	23	24	25	26	27	28	29	30	1	2	3	4	5	6	7		JULY
OCTOBER	1	2	3	4	5	6	7	8	9	10	11	12	13	14	15	16	17	18	19	20	21	22	23	24	25	26	27	28	29	30	31	OCTOBER
JULY	8	9	10	11	12	13	14	15	16	17	18	19	20	21	22	23	24	25	26	27	28	29	30	31	1	2	3	4	5	6	7	AUGUST
NOVEMBER	1	2	3	4	5	6	7	8	9	10	11	12	13	14	15	16	17	18	19	20	21	22	23	24	25	26	27	28	29	30		NOVEMBER
AUGUST	8	9	10	11	12	13	14	15	16	17	18	19	20	21	22	23	24	25	26	27	28	29	30	31	1	2	3	4	5	6		SEPTEMBER
DECEMBER	1	2	3	4	5	6	7	8	9	10	11	12	13	14	15	16	17	18	19	20	21	22	23	24	25	26	27	28	29	30	31	DECEMBER
SEPTEMBER	7	8	9	10	11	12	13	14	15	16	17	18	19	20	21	22	23	24	25	26	27	28	29	30	1	2	3	4	5	6	7	OCTOBER

cally implies "completion," as represented by the seven days of Creation. Seven times forty is two hundred and eighty — a symbol of the complete preparation of a human being from before conception to birth.

NOTES

1. B. Landau, *Essential Human Anatomy and Physiology* (Scott, Foresman and Co.), p. 699.
2. L. Zacharias, W.M. Rand, R.J. Wurtman, "A Prospective Study of Sexual Development and Growth in American Girls: the Statistics of Menarche," *Obstetric Gynecological Survey* 31:325, 1976; *see also Niddah* 45a.
3. Rashi, *Yoma* 47a; *see* Hebrew appendix.
4. L. Speroff, R.H. Glass, et al., *Clinical Gynecologic Endocrinology and Fertility*, 3rd ed. (Baltimore: Williams and Wilkins, 1983).
5. A. Pilliteri, *Maternal-Newborn Nursing* (Boston: Little, Brown & Co., 1981), p. 145.
6. *Niddah* 38a.
7. W.D. Todd, D.F. Tapley, eds., *Columbia University College of Physicians and Surgeons' Complete Guide to Pregnancy* (New York: Crown Publishers), p. 66.
8. *Sotah* 2a.
9. Rama, *Yoreh De'ah* 242:31; *see* Shach, 49.

3 | Life inside the Womb

*A light burns above [the fetus'] head and
he looks and sees from one end of the
world to the other. He is taught all the
Torah from beginning to end, and there is
no time of life when a person enjoys
greater happiness. For it is said, 'Oh that
I were as the months of old as in the days
when God watched over me.'*

NIDDAH 30b

From fertilization until birth, the fetus is dependent upon certain components to sustain its life.

The PLACENTA is the channel of supply between the uterine wall on the maternal side and the umbilical cord on the fetal side. It is round and flat, 8 in. (20 cm.) in diameter and 1 in. (2.5 cm.) thick, weighing approximately one-sixth of the baby's weight at term.

Much like the roots of a plant, the placenta draws substances necessary to sustain fetal life from the mother's blood. It provides nutritional, respiratory, excretory and endocrine (hormonal) functions for the fetus, in addition to serving as a screen to protect the fetus by neutralizing certain drugs and diseases. Every enzyme known to exist in biology has been found in the placenta.[1]

The UMBILICAL CORD contains two arteries and one vein. In most cases arteries deliver fresh, oxygenated blood throughout the body, and the veins transport carbon dioxide back to the heart. Paradoxically, through

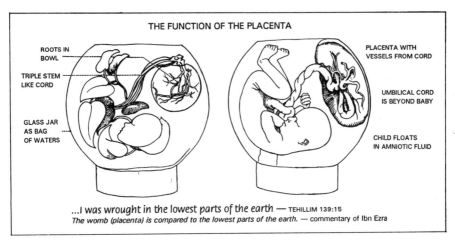

THE FUNCTION OF THE PLACENTA

ROOTS IN BOWL

TRIPLE STEM LIKE CORD

GLASS JAR AS BAG OF WATERS

PLACENTA WITH VESSELS FROM CORD

UMBILICAL CORD IS BEYOND BABY

CHILD FLOATS IN AMNIOTIC FLUID

...I was wrought in the lowest parts of the earth — TEHILLIM 139:15
The womb (placenta) is compared to the lowest parts of the earth. — commentary of Ibn Ezra

the umbilical cord, unoxygenated blood is directed back to the placenta through the arteries, while one umbilical vein supplies pure oxygenated blood enriched with nutrients from the placenta. The umbilical cord appears to contain no nerve supply and is cut at birth without any discomfort to either baby or mother.[2]

Within the uterus, the fetus is surrounded by the FETAL SAC, a double-walled capsule filled with fluid. The outer membrane (wall) is called the chorion and the inner membrane the amnion. The fetus and the amniotic fluid are held within the amniotic membrane.

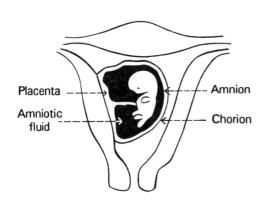

Placenta

Amniotic fluid

Amnion

Chorion

AMNIOTIC FLUID is clear, pale and straw-colored. At term, the amniotic sac holds 17-51 oz. (500-1500 ml.) of fluid. Although amniotic fluid is 99% water, it also contains many elements which, upon close examination, reveal vital information about the baby's condition.

The baby is protected and cushioned throughout the pregnancy as he floats in his warm, fluid world. The

Gemara describes the embryo within the mother's womb as a nut floating in a bowl of water. Should someone put his finger upon it, it would sink on one side or the other.[3] A pregnant woman can feel this sensation for herself. Lying flat on her back, she can gently apply pressure to different areas of the abdomen, causing the baby to float away from her touch.

Nine months may seem like a long time to wait to embrace and welcome our newborn into the world. Yet, once we understand the magnitude and intri- **Fetal Development** cacy of fetal growth and development, nine months may seem inadequate. This awareness can only deepen our appreciation of Hashem's handiwork in forming a human being.

The embryo begins as a group of indistinguishable cells which separate into three layers: the ectoderm, the endoderm and the mesoderm. These three layers form the basis of the distinctive body systems. From the ectoderm (outer layer) the nervous system, skin, hair, nails, sense organs, and mucous membranes of the mouth and anus will develop. The endoderm (inner layer) develops into the lining of the gastrointestinal tract, the respiratory tract, tonsils, thyroid and thymus glands, and the bladder and urethra. The mesoderm (middle layer) forms the supportive structures of the body (tissue, bones, cartilage, muscle, and tendons), kidneys and ureters, the reproductive system, and the blood cells.

Our Sages teach us that the formation of the fetus begins with the head.[4] Modern medical research has confirmed this fact, describing fetal development as proceeding in a head-to-tail direction, with the head developing first.

FETAL DEVELOPMENT AND PRAYER

The Talmud advises us how to formulate our prayers in relation to the development of the fetus:

During the first three days of conception one should pray that the pregnancy be accepted by the body.

From three to forty days after conception one may pray for a specific determination of the sex of the child. An example of the ability to influence the sex of the fetus through prayer is demonstrated by the story of Leah. The Torah explains why each of Yaakov's sons was given his specific name, yet no reason is given for the name Dinah. The Gemara explains that Leah pronounced judgment (*din*) against herself, saying, "If this child also is a male, I will have produced seven males, and each of the handmaidens two. My sister Rachel would only be left one son, and would not even be the equal of the handmaidens." Therefore she prayed to Hashem that the child she was carrying be female, and the sex of the child was indeed changed. The Talmud concludes that Leah's prayer took place before the fortieth day of her pregnancy, since the sex of the fetus would have been determined by the fortieth day and afterwards her prayer would have been in vain.[5]

From forty days to three months one should pray that the child not suffer from any deformity.

From three months to six months it is proper to offer prayers that one not miscarry.

From six months to nine months one should pray that the baby be delivered safely.[6]

Gestational Development

THE VERY BEGINNING

The fetus progresses rapidly from a cellular mass to a being of distinctive physical features. Following implantation (5-7 days after conception) the placenta and umbilical cord begin to develop. From the region of the head, a single tube forms, eventually becoming the heart. During this early embryonic period, the respiratory and digestive tracts exist as a single tube, and one week later the two systems begin to divide. At this time the lung buds also begin to appear. During the third and fourth week the formation of the nervous system and sense organs has already begun.

Your Pregnancy at a Glance

It's only about two weeks since conception. You may not even have missed your period — but you suspect something is "different."

FOUR WEEKS

By the time four weeks have passed from the woman's last menstrual cycle, the head comprises about a third of the entire embryo. A single-chambered heart is beating, and an immature neural plate, the foundation of the central nervous system, is evident. The umbilical cord is already functional, transporting oxygen, carbon dioxide and nutrients to and from the placenta.
☞ The embryo is less than 1/10 of an inch (2 mm.) in size.

EIGHT WEEKS

At eight weeks the baby is no longer referred to as an embryo but as a fetus. Pregnancy can already be confirmed by an ultrasound. Eight weeks also marks the completion of "organogenesis" — the formation of the fetal organs.

The heart chambers have been divided. Facial features are more discernible, which gives the fetus a more human-like appearance. Legs, arms, fingers, toes, elbows, and knees have developed. External genitalia are present, but the sex is not clear. In fact, the fetus has all the components to develop into either a male or female, but does not acquire definitive male or female characteristics until the seventh week of development.[7] The Talmud tells us that the fetus develops into either male or female in the first 41 days of life.[8] This parallels our potential for prayer to determine the sex of the child until the fortieth day after conception.
☞ The fetus is half an inch (1.3 cm.) in length and weighs about 1/30 oz. (1 gr.).

You've confirmed your pregnancy with a blood test or urinalysis. It's very exciting — your own secret to share with those closest to you. You may feel a bit queasy, but try to maintain your regular schedule.

TWELVE WEEKS

Twelve weeks marks the end of the first of three trimesters (3-month periods). The placenta is now fully mature and functional.[9] It is thus resistant to most teratogens (drugs, diseases, pollutants, or radiation that can cause deformities, retar-

Now you see your stomach starting to swell. You're a bit tired — those afternoon naps are a lifesaver. You've most probably heard

dation or even death, God forbid). During the first eight weeks of intrauterine life, the fetus is especially vulnerable, and the specific organs developing at the time of contact with a teratogen would be harmed. We can now understand *Chazal*'s advice to pray for the completeness of the child during this time. (See Chapter 6 on Safe Pregnancy Guidelines.)

At this stage, the brain and spinal cord are already well-developed, and the kidneys have begun to excrete urine. Though there is fetal movement, the mother cannot feel it yet. The heartbeat can be heard at the pre-natal check-up.

Nail beds are forming on fingers and toes. Tooth buds are present. Male and female are distinguishable by outward appearance, and the baby's sex can be determined by ultrasound.

Rav Simlai says: What does the fetus look like inside its mother? It is curled up with its arms at its sides. Its hands rest on its two temples, its two elbows on its two legs, and its two heels against its buttocks. Its head lies between its knees.[10]

☞ The fetus is 2.6 in. (6.5 cm.) in length, and weighs 1 3/4 oz. (20 gr.).

your baby's heartbeat at the prenatal checkup — it's real!

SIXTEEN WEEKS

Fine downy hair (lanugo) appears on the fetus, serving as insulation for body heat. By swallowing amniotic fluid and urinating, the fetus produces the continual circulation of amniotic fluid through his body and the fetal sac. Meconium, the fetal waste product, starts to accumulate in the intestines. The eyes, ears, and nose are in their final positions.

☞ The fetus is 4.4 in. (11 cm.) in length and weighs 4 oz. (124 gr.).

You're feeling much better now that the nausea has passed. They say that the second trimester is easier. You've chosen some maternity clothes — so pack away the old things. Try to eat healthily and exercise.

TWENTY WEEKS

By now, the mother will have felt her baby move for the first time. The first sensation of fetal movement is called "quickening," and feels like butterflies or gas bubbles.

Everyone can tell by now that you're "in the family way." You may start to feel your baby's

Throughout the second half of pregnancy, fetal movements will be a constant reminder that the baby is healthy and developing.

☞ The length of the fetus is 6 in. (15 cm.) and weighs 8 oz. (248 gr.).

movements — little butterflies in your stomach. You've got quite an appetite, but try to avoid overeating.

TWENTY-FOUR WEEKS

Twenty-four weeks marks the end of the second trimester. The fetus' skin is red and wrinkled and covered by a cheesy-white substance (vernix caseosa) which protects and lubricates the fetal skin. Eyebrows and lashes have developed and the eyelids are open. Maternal antibodies, protection against illness, are being transferred to the fetus. The fetus is considered viable with intensive care if born after 24 weeks or 22 oz. (601 gr.).[11]

☞ The fetus' length (from head to toe) is 8 in. (20 cm.) and weighs 1 1/3 lb. (600 gr.).

You definitely feel the baby moving by now. When you lie on your left side, he becomes very active, reminding you of the miracle growing inside you. It's nice that people get up to offer you a seat on the bus.

TWENTY-EIGHT WEEKS

The fetal lungs are maturing and producing an enzyme needed to prevent the lungs from collapsing when exhaling (surfactant). One of the major dangers for a preterm baby is respiratory distress syndrome (RDS). In these cases a respirator is needed to help the baby breathe. With God's help, medical technology is constantly improving and offering greater hope for premature infants.

☞ A 28-week-old fetus is 14.4 in. (37 cm.) from head to toe and weighs 2 1/2 lb. (1.1 kg.).

Bending down isn't quite as easy as it used to be. Now you're entering the third trimester — nine months isn't such a long time after all. You've enrolled in a childbirth preparation course.

THIRTY-TWO WEEKS

The fetus acquires subcutaneous fat deposits which change the skin from red to flesh color. Research has shown that the fetus not only reacts to touch but is also aware and reacts to sounds outside the mother's body.[12] His hearing ability is not surprising, as the inner ear is already well developed by the middle of the pregnancy. As

Sometimes your stomach feels so high that it's hard to catch your breath. You may also have heartburn. Eating smaller, more frequent meals and sleeping with extra pillows is a

a matter of fact, parents have reported success in calming a fussy newborn by playing a recording of the human heartbeat or ocean surf, which is reminiscent of the rhythmic heartbeat of the mother and the waves of amniotic fluid which surrounded the fetus for so many months.

☞ The fetus is 17 in. (43 cm.) in length and weighs 3 1/2-4 lb. (1.6-1.8 kg.).

big help. It's a good idea to check in a full-length mirror now and again to make sure your dress is long enough and your knees aren't showing!

THIRTY-SIX WEEKS

Upon reaching thirty-six weeks, the fetus begins to store supplies of iron, carbohydrates and calcium, which he will need for the first few months of life. He is looking plumper and has assumed the position he will be in at the time of delivery. At any time during the third trimester the mother may even feel her baby shifting to his final birth position. She may feel a sudden increase of activity or a few unusually strong kicks, but there is no need for concern as long as she continues to feel regular fetal movement.

☞ Length is 18 in. (46 cm.) and weight is from 5-6 lb. (2.2-2.7 kg.).

You've hit the home stretch — the last month. Prepare your travel bag and be ready any time.

FORTY WEEKS

At forty weeks the baby is fully developed and considered "full term." Lanugo hair disappears. In a male, both testes should have descended into the scrotum. Nails project beyond the ends of the fingers and toes. The intestines contain meconium, a greenish-black waste substance which will be passed soon after delivery.

☞ Average length for a mature newborn is 20 in. (50 cm.) and weight is 7-7.5 lb. (3.4 kg.).

B'SHA'AH TOVAH!

The fetus must undergo one more crucial step in his development before he enters the world, one which is probably not recorded in other pregnancy books. The Talmud says: "The fetus does not leave the womb until he takes an oath, promising to be always righteous and never wicked...Always remember that the Holy One, Blessed Be He, is pure, His angels are pure and that the soul which He gave you is pure."[13]

At this point the baby is ready. It is time to be born.

NOTES

1. M. Myles, *Textbook for Midwives* (Edinburgh: Churchill Livingstone, 1981), p. 45.
2. A. Pilliteri, *Maternal-Newborn Nursing* (Boston: Little, Brown & Co.), p. 490.
3. *Niddah* 31a.
4. *Yoma* 85a; *see* Hebrew appendix.
5. The Gemara offers an alternative conclusion. In consideration of Leah's righteousness and the special circumstances, God miraculously changed the sex of the fetus even after the fortieth day.
6. *Berachos* 60a.
7. T.W. Sadler, *Medical Embryology* (Baltimore: Williams & Wilkins, 1990), p. 271.
8. *Niddah* 30a.
9. During the first trimester, the corpus luteum, the portion of the ovarian follicle which remains after releasing the ovum, supports the pregnancy until the placenta is fully developed.
10. *Niddah* 30b.
11. A. Pilliteri, *Maternal-Newborn Nursing* (Boston: Little, Brown & Co.), p. 161.
12. *The Developing Human: Clinically Oriented Embryology*, 2nd ed. (Phildelphia: Saunders, 1977).
13. *Niddah* 30b.

4 | Prenatal Care

A person toils with his two hands and
Hashem sends His blessing.
TANCHUMA, VAYETZE 13

Once pregnancy has been confirmed, the mother-to-be must take special care of herself and her unborn baby. She should schedule her first prenatal checkup as soon as she discovers that she is pregnant.

Faith in the Almighty or in the Doctor? Some God-fearing Jews ask, Why should I go to the doctor for checkups if *Hakadosh Baruch Hu* controls everything in my life? Isn't it more appropriate to pray to Hashem for good health rather than rely on the wisdom of mortal men?

This question has its origins in Rabbinic literature. The Rambam admonishes those who say that a sick person who goes to a doctor to be healed is demonstrating a lack of faith in Hashem. According to the Rambam, this compares to saying that one who eats bread in order to relieve the "disease" called hunger is also demonstrating a lack of faith, because the person should have prayed to the Almighty and relied on Him to cure the hunger.[1]

The Ramban, on the other hand, says that the *tzaddikim* did not go to doctors, but to the Prophets.[2] In other words, physical ailments can be cured by strengthening our spirituality.

The *halachah* clearly follows the Rambam, determining that one should go to doctors not only to *cure* illness but also to *prevent* it. Even the Ramban would agree that only a select group of very pious individuals could rely on their spirituality and refrain from visiting a doctor. Most people are not on that spiritual plane, however, and modern medicine, while not perfect, is generally effective. The *Birkei Yosef* writes, "Today one should not rely on a miracle. A sick person is required to act according to the ways of the world and call a doctor. And no one has permission to deviate from the custom of the world."[3] The *Shevet Yehudah* says, "A sick person is strongly obligated to seek out a good doctor and medicines. And whoever is lax in doing so and relies on a miracle, saying that Hashem will send his cure, is considered foolish. He is being negligent with his own body, and in the future he will have to face judgment for doing so."[4]

This does not contradict our faith in the Almighty. Of course we believe that our good health is in the hands of Hashem. Medicine and the advice of doctors are merely the tools that we must use in seeking a cure. Together with this, we must also pray to Hashem that the medicine and treatment will be beneficial to us.

Another question is sometimes asked: If Hashem made us ill, wouldn't it be considered interference with God's will if we cure the illness? Hashem obviously has a reason for making us sick.

The following *Midrash* provides an answer: Rabbi Yishmael, Rabbi Akiva, and a companion were walking along together in Jerusalem. They met a sick person, who asked them, "Rabbis, how can I be healed?" The Sages gave him medical advice that would cure him.

The man asked, "Who made me ill?" And they answered, "Hashem." The sick man then questioned their interference with the will of God.

The Sages responded by asking the man his occupation. He showed them his scythe and replied that he was a farmer. The Rabbis then asked, "Who created the vineyard?" And the farmer responded that Hashem had created the vineyard. "Then aren't you interfering with something that is not yours?" asked the Rabbis. "Hashem created it and you are taking the fruits." The farmer replied that if he were not to use his scythe to clear his land, or if he didn't plow, fertilize, or weed, then nothing would grow.

The Sages then admonished the farmer, referring to *Tehillim*: "As for man, his days are like grass." A man is like a tree which requires the farmer's care. If the farmer were not to weed and plow, the tree would not grow. And even once it grows, it still requires irrigation and fertilization. So it is with the human body. The medicine can be compared to fertilizer, and the doctor can be compared to the farmer.[5]

THE CORRECT BALANCE

Those who rely on a miracle for their good health are considered foolish. Those who think their good health depends on modern medicine and does not ultimately lie in the hands of God are nonbelievers. We must choose between the two extremes and find the Golden Path.

The Chazon Ish related to this dilemma in the following letter:

> Concerning myself, I consider the physical effort to maintain good health to be both an obligation and a mitzvah. It is one of the requirements dictated by the Creator for self-perfection. It is recorded that *Amora'im* [Rabbis of the Talmudic period] went to doctors of other nations to become cured. It is evident that much of the plant and animal life serves medicinal purposes. Also, gates of wisdom were created for all to contemplate and achieve understanding. However, the ways of the Divine may bypass natural laws as well as the efforts man puts into using them. What is needed is the correct balance. Deviation from the true path is not acceptable — whether it is to rely on the level of faith which I have honestly reached, or to believe too much in the natural order.[6]

The correct balance between human effort and faith in the Divine is an essential of Judaism. This does not apply only to matters of health, but to all aspects of our lives. There is no contradiction. These efforts complement one another. On the one hand, our Sages tell us that a *talmid chacham* should not live in a city that does not have a doctor.[7] On the other hand, they also tell us that when the Jewish people raise their eyes to Heaven and submit in their hearts to Hashem, they will be healed.[8]

Prenatal Checkups

The person caring for you may be a private physician, nurse practitioner, or certified midwife. Routine prenatal checkups are carried out in the doctor's office, or the community or hospital clinic. There are standard requirements for prenatal exams during the various stages of pregnancy. Initially, prenatal checkups are scheduled once every month to six weeks, but as the due date draws near, checkups are scheduled on a more frequent basis.

At your first prenatal checkup, your doctor will review your medical history and current health status. He will also give you a thorough checkup, including both a breast and pelvic (internal) examination.

Pelvic Exam

After pregnancy is officially diagnosed, the pelvic exam is especially significant for its ability to reveal any potential problems. It consists of two parts. At first, the doctor examines the vagina and cervix with the aid of a speculum. The speculum holds the vagina open in order to enable better visualization of the cervix and vaginal walls. At this point the doctor may perform a cervical smear (PAP test). A cotton swab is wiped across the cervix, removing a few cells for microscopic analysis. This test can detect early cervical changes which may precede the development of cancer. The speculum will only be in place for about one minute, and is not uncomfortable if you are relaxed.

The second part is the bi-manual (internal) exam. In order to indirectly feel the uterus and ovaries, the doctor inserts two fingers into the vagina, pushing up against the cervix, while simultaneously pressing down on the abdomen. By ascertaining that the uterus is enlarged, this exam serves as a further confirmation of pregnancy. It also rules out any structural abnormalities of the pelvis, vagina and cervix that could interfere with pregnancy or delivery. Cervical dilation is also evaluated during the bi-manual examination.

The pelvic exam is generally not repeated during prenatal visits unless there are suspected complications. One need not fear that either exam (during the initial visit or during a regular gynecological checkup) induces the *niddah* status. It is not necessary to do a *bedikah* or even to ask a Rav, unless there are particular problems such as bleeding, pain or contractions.[9]

Urinalysis A sample of urine will be taken in the clinic, and it will be analyzed on-the-spot by means of a special reagent strip (Clinistix). The results will show if the levels of glucose or protein in the urine are too high, indicating the possibility of diabetes, urinary tract infection or high blood pressure.

A laboratory urinalysis will also be performed at the beginning of the pregnancy. It will ascertain the levels of certain electrolytes as well as the sterility of the urine, ensuring that no infectious bacteria are present. This urinalysis may be repeated if a urinary tract infection is suspected or just as a matter of routine.

Blood Pressure Blood pressure may fluctuate during pregnancy. If it becomes low, the doctor will encourage you to increase your fluid intake. Even though high blood pressure is most often caused by nervousness, anxiety or pain, it must be strictly monitored, as it may also be a symptom of more serious conditions. See Chapter 5 on Body Changes for a more detailed explanation of high blood pressure.

Weight Weight gain is also carefully recorded during prenatal visits. Pregnancy is not the time to diet, because both mother and baby need the added weight for proper development and good health. Any sudden weight gain or loss may be an indication of illness.

The average expected weight gain in pregnancy is 25-30 lb., or 11.3-13.1 kg. This may seem like a great deal of weight to gain. However, if you gain by eating properly (as described in Chapter 8 on Nutrition), the weight will be distributed where it is needed. Women who were underweight before becoming pregnant can expect to gain more, and those who were overweight may naturally gain less.

Distribution of Weight Gain		
	pounds	kilograms
fetus	7.0	3.1
placenta	1.5	.6
amniotic fluid	2.0	.9
uterus	2.5	1.1
blood volume	3.5	1.5
breasts	1.5-3.0	.6-1.3
body fluid	8.0	3.6
TOTAL	26.0-27.5	11.4-12.1

Weight gain during the first three months is slight, about 3 lb. or 1-2 kg. Being nauseous during the first trimester might even cause you to lose weight. During the second and third trimester you can expect to gain approximately 1 lb. (about half a kg.) a week.

Weight gain varies with each pregnancy. You will probably buy your first maternity clothes around the end of the first trimester, and you may need to add a few items along the way, especially with the change of seasons during the nine months of your pregnancy. In addition to clothing, it is most likely that you will require larger size bras by the end of the first trimester. Breast growth should stabilize by the 32nd to 36th week, and then you can buy a nursing bra which will serve until the end of the pregnancy and after delivery.

Edema   Edema is the retention of fluids in the body. The doctor will examine your legs and ankles for edema by pressing and trying to indent the skin with his fingers. A slight swelling around the ankles is considered normal toward the end of pregnancy, but excessive fluid retention in the legs, hands and face warrants further medical investigation.

Abdominal Examination   At each prenatal visit, the abdomen will be externally examined to assess the growth of the uterus and the size of the fetus. The highest point of the uterus (the fundus) is measured, indicating the growth of the baby. At week 12, the uterus has risen to just above the pubic bone; at week 20, to the level of the navel; and at week 28, the fundus can be felt just below the sternum.

The outline of the baby is perceived by means of gentle palpation. The experienced caregiver can thus determine the fetus' size, position and the location of the fetus' head in relation to the mother's pelvis.

An electronic instrument called a doppler or doptone has in most cases replaced the manual fetal stethoscope. It is used to listen to the fetal heart rate. It is always exciting and reassuring to hear your baby's heartbeat at each checkup and to know that he's doing okay.

Blood Tests   Blood tests are an important part of routine prenatal care. At the beginning of every pregnancy, the following blood tests are done:

BLOOD TYPE (A, B, AB, or O)

RH FACTOR (positive or negative)

VDRL (a blood test which screens syphilis)

HEMOGLOBIN/HEMATOCRIT (test for anemia)

FASTING BLOOD GLUCOSE (blood is taken in the morning, when no food has been eaten since midnight; tests blood sugar to rule out diabetes).

Another blood test which is considered standard is the test for rubella antibodies (resistance to German measles). One may have acquired immunity either by having the disease or by being immunized. German measles during pregnancy can have a disastrous effect on the fetus. It is therefore incumbent upon every woman to have this test done at the beginning of her child-bearing years. If she is not immune, she should have a vaccination against rubella after she gives birth. Pregnancy must be avoided for three months after receiving the rubella vaccine. A Rav should be consulted regarding birth control options.

The results of these initial blood tests will determine what additional blood tests will be required throughout your pregnancy. Some tests are repeated on a routine basis, such as the hemoglobin/hematocrit level, which is tested again in the second and third trimester.

If the mother's blood glucose was elevated, additional testing will be needed to monitor the possibility of gestational diabetes (diabetes induced by pregnancy). The postprandial (after eating) glucose test is taken two hours after she has eaten a carbohydrate-rich meal. This blood test is routinely done at 28 weeks for any woman who has a family history of diabetes.

The oral glucose tolerance test (OGTT) is a more comprehensive blood analysis. After drinking 50 gr. of liquid glucose, blood is taken at 30 minutes, 1 hour, 2 hours, and then 3 hours to evaluate the body's response to glucose. (See Chapter 5 for a more thorough discussion of diabetes in pregnancy.)

The Rh Negative Mother

If the mother's blood type (Rh factor) is negative, she will be tested for Rh antibodies at 18-20 weeks and monthly thereafter until delivery. Rh is an abbreviation for rhesus factor, an antigen present in red blood cells. Most people are Rh positive, and only about 17% are Rh negative.

The complications of Rh incompatibility will only occur in a case where the mother is Rh negative and the father is Rh positive. When an Rh-positive fetus begins to grow inside an Rh-negative mother, her body reacts as if it has been invaded by a foreign agent or disease. Antibodies are produced to attack the invading substance, which can cause the destruction of fetal red blood cells.

During pregnancy, the blood of the baby and the mother generally do not mix. Mixing is more likely to occur during delivery, when a small amount (about 2cc.) of fetal blood enters the maternal circulation. From this point on, the Rh-negative mother produces antibodies against the Rh-positive antigen. These antibodies can be deployed against an Rh-positive fetus in subsequent pregnancies.

In our day and age, Rh incompatibility can be prevented. It is now common practice for every Rh-negative woman to receive an Anti-D immunization in the 28th week of pregnancy to insure against the formation of antibodies. Although the risk of developing Rh incompatibility is much less in a first pregnancy, Anti-D is still given to Rh-negative women as an extra precaution. Another Anti-D injection is administered 72 hours after the birth of an Rh-positive baby to an RH-negative woman, or after any miscarriage or abortion.

Other Diagnostic Examinations   In addition to routine diagnostic examinations, other diagnostic tests are done to enhance the quality of prenatal care.

AFP (ALPHA FETOPROTEIN) is a test of the mother's blood to rule out fetal malformations. It is usually done at 16 weeks gestation. There is no risk to mother or baby. An elevated serum AFP may indicate nervous system defects (such as spina bifida), and a low serum AFP may indicate the possibility of Down's Syndrome (mongolism). Since the results demonstrate only a ratio of risk for a potential problem, an amniocentesis is always needed to confirm any specific defect. Because the test results only serve to give a woman peace of mind by ruling out dreaded defects, AFP is considered optional. On the other hand, this test is considered controversial and there are a large number of false positives which only serve to increase maternal anxiety. A woman should consider her motives before testing for AFP and what reaction she might have in the event of disheartening results. AFP is basically a first-step screening for high-risk pregnancies. A Rav need not be consulted before this optional blood test.[10]

AMNIOCENTESIS is the aspiration of a sample of amniotic fluid for analysis. The amniotic fluid contains fetal cells, which, when examined, can reveal detailed information about the condition of the fetus. Amniocentesis is most often performed at 16 weeks to detect chromosomal defects (for example, Tay-Sachs). Later in pregnancy this test is done to verify lung maturity if a premature birth is imminent.

Most medical authorities recommend a routine amniocentesis in women over 35 years old, because of the increased risk of Down's Syndrome.[11] Women who have a history of genetic disorders or who have received abnormal Alpha Fetoprotein results will also be encouraged to undergo amniocentesis.

The amniocentesis takes about twenty minutes to perform. The doctor usually administers a local anesthetic, then inserts a long, thin needle through the abdomen into the amniotic sac, and withdraws a small amount of fluid. The woman is continuously monitored by an ultrasound to ensure the

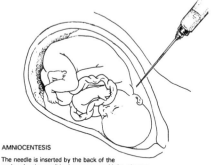

AMNIOCENTESIS

The needle is inserted by the back of the neck or by the small body parts to avoid the placenta.

successful placement of the needle. After the amniocentesis, the fetus is again examined by ultrasound to confirm his well-being.

It takes two to four weeks to obtain the results of the

laboratory analysis. It should be noted that there is a slight risk of miscarriage (.5%) whenever an amniocentesis is performed.[12]

Some *poskim* have determined that an amniocentesis which is performed for the purpose of diagnosing possible birth defects is forbidden.[13] In some specific cases, however, *poskim* have allowed it.[14] It is, therefore, clearly forbidden to undergo amniocentesis without prior consultation with a Rav.

Yet an amniocentesis which is performed to evaluate lung maturity at the end of pregnancy is unquestionably halachically allowed. It is usually performed in cases where the baby's welfare is in doubt, and an induced premature delivery is being considered. Knowing if the fetal lungs are mature might be the deciding factor in whether or not delivery should be induced.

A relatively new test, CHORIONIC VILLUS SAMPLING (CVS), can detect birth defects as early as week 8-12 of pregnancy. Results are available within forty-eight hours.

This procedure also lasts about twenty minutes. A thin tube (catheter) is introduced into the cervix or through the abdomen, and a small sample of tissue is removed from the developing placenta. Ultrasound guidance is continuous during testing. Though CVS is performed throughout the world with increasing frequency, there are claims of resultant limb anomalies.[15] Research continues and some medical centers have begun to restrict the use of CVS to 10 weeks gestation and beyond.[16] There is also a greater risk of miscarriage (1-2%) than with amniocentesis.[17] A Rav must be consulted before undergoing this examination.[18]

ULTRASOUND (or sonography) has become a routine diagnostic tool in pregnancy. Intermittent sound waves are projected toward the uterus. The sound waves bounce off the baby's bones and tissues, and the echoes are converted into images, which are displayed on a television screen. Various shades of light and dark reflect the thickness of the tissues.

In over 25 years of use worldwide, no harmful effects have been associated with the use of ultrasound.[19]

The American College of Obstetricians and Gynecologists recommends ultrasound to assess the overall condition of pregnancy only when certain factors are present, for example:

— the size of the fetus does not correspond to the calculated age of pregnancy

— the woman has not been under proper medical guidance throughout pregnancy

— or if a previous child was born with malformations.[20]

Opinions vary as to how many ultrasounds need to be done during pregnancy.

According to Dr. Chaim Yaffe, Head of Obstetrics and Gynecology at Bikur Cholim Hospital in Jerusalem, a common practice in Europe and Israel is for two ultrasounds to be performed during pregnancy: one ultrasound at 20 weeks and the second at 33 weeks.

The reasons are:

1. to accurately estimate the gestational age of the fetus;

2. to diagnose the presence of multiple fetuses (twins);

3. to observe the condition and location of the placenta (if implanted too close to the cervix, special followup is essential);

4. to serve as a reference for any potential disruptions in growth and development that might occur at a later stage; and

5. to rule out malformations.

Additional ultrasounds are generally requested if any specific problems are suspected.

There are cases where early detection in utero of treatable malformations, of the kidneys or in the digestive tract for example, has saved the baby's life. Otherwise the problem might go undetected at birth, only to be diagnosed when it is too late for treatment.

Ultrasound has proven to be a valuable, non-invasive aid in providing comprehensive prenatal care.

ELECTRONIC MONITORING affords simultaneous measurement of the fetal heart rate and uterine activity (contractions). As the monitor is often an integral part of prenatal care and of labor and delivery, it is beneficial to understand how it works. There are basically two variations of electronic monitoring: external or internal.

EXTERNAL METHOD

The method used most is external monitoring. The equipment consists of two belts with one round transducer on each belt. The first belt is applied to the most protruding part of the abdomen (the uterine fundus). This transducer records contractions. Uterine contractions register from 20, indicating a relaxed uterus, to 80-100 during a strong contraction.

The second belt is placed on the lower half of the abdomen, either to the left or right, and it records the fetal heart rate. The transducer measures sound waves which are radiated through a clear, non-staining jelly. The sound waves of the baby's heartbeat are projected toward the transducer through his back. It may, therefore, be difficult to locate and monitor the heartbeat if the mother is obese, if there is too much amniotic fluid (polyhydramnios), or if the fetus is lying in a position where his back is inaccessible.

Two numbers — the uterine contractions and the fetal heart rate — are illuminated on the monitor.

When using an external monitor, the registered strength of the contraction is not totally accurate. The most valuable information that the external monitor offers is the length and frequency of the contractions and the correlation of the fetal heart rate. Just as our heart rate fluctuates depending upon physical activity, the same is true for the baby in utero. These fluctuations in heart rate are an indication of your baby's well-being.

By week 34, it is possible to monitor accelerations in

the fetal heart rate during physical activity or uterine contractions. At least two accelerations normally occur within the span of twenty minutes. One expected variation occurs when the fetus sleeps. Then the fetal heart rate is unvarying, with no accelerations or decelerations.

For best results, it is recommended to eat and drink within an hour before you are monitored. This "wakes up" the baby so his true heartbeat can be measured. Lying on your left side will also elicit optimal activity in your baby. A normal fetal heart rate is 120-160 beats per minute. When the fetal heart rate is measured externally, any movement on the part of the mother or baby can result in "losing" the heartbeat. Although you may find this quite alarming, within seconds you or the baby will settle down, and the monitor will register the heartbeat.

The doptone or doppler functions in a way similar to the external fetal heart monitor. It is a small, portable fetal heart monitor, which is generally used during prenatal checkups or for a quick assessment of the fetal heart rate during labor.

INTERNAL METHOD

When more precise monitoring is required, the internal method is employed. The waters must be broken before the fetal heart rate or uterine contractions can be monitored internally. To measure uterine contractions, a long thin tube (catheter) is painlessly introduced through the cervix, and is set alongside the baby in the uterus. The strength and frequency of uterine contractions can thus be more accurately measured by means of pressure changes in the amniotic fluid.

The baby's heartbeat is internally measured by use of a spiral electrode attached to the baby's scalp. After delivery, the mother may notice a small red scratch on the baby's scalp, which will disappear within a few days.

In addition to being more accurate, internal monitoring allows for greater freedom of movement. Although the mother must still lie in bed, she can turn from side to side without the monitor losing the heartbeat. The pace of labor and delivery are not affected by the use of internal monitoring, and there is virtually no risk.

Prenatal care involves a team: the doctor, the clinic staff and you. During this period, it is important to be comfortable enough with the team to communicate your questions and feelings. Having confidence in your health care will give you a more positive, worry-free pregnancy.

NOTES

1. Rambam, *Mishnah Pesachim* 4:10.
2. Ramban, *Vayikra* 26:11.
3. *Birkei Yosef, Yoreh De'ah* 336:2.
4. *Shevet Yehudah, Shulchan Aruch, Yoreh De'ah* 336.
5. *Midrash Shemuel, parashah* 4.
6. Chazon Ish, *Letters*, vol. I, letter 136.
7. *Sanhedrin* 17b.
8. *Rosh Hashanah* 29a. Concerning visits to the doctor in regard to *yichud*, consult your *Rav*. See *Iggros Moshe, Even Ha-Ezer*, vol. IV, ch. 65,1.
9. *See* Hebrew appendix.
10. Heard from R. Mordechai Eliyahu.
11. C. Stern, *Human Genetics* (San Francisco: Freeman, 1973).
12. H.R. Barber, D.H. Fields, S.A. Kaufman *O.B.-GYN Procedures* (Philadelphia: Lippincott Co., 1990), p. 73.
13. *Iggros Moshe, Choshen Mishpat*, vol. II, ch. 71.
14. *Tzitz Eliezer*, vol. XIV, 101.
15. B.K. Burton, L.I. Burd, C. Schulz, *Obstetrics and Gynecology*, 79:726-30, 1992.
16. P.A. Boyd, P. Chamberlin, H.V. Firth, et al., *Lancet*, 337:762-63, 1991.
17. D.F. Tapley, W.D. Todd, eds., *The Columbia University Complete Guide to Pregnancy* (New York: Crown, 1988), p. 151.
18. Heard from R. Mordechai Eliyahu.
19. J. Drukners, R. Knuppel, *High Risk Pregnancy* (Philadelphia: W.B. Saunders, 1986), p. 57.
20. D.F. Tapley, W.D. Todd, eds., *The Columbia University Complete Guide to Pregnancy* (New York: Crown Publishers, Inc.), p. 151.

5 | Body Changes

The word Torah is written in feminine form — the reason being that Torah brings a person to the path of life.
MAHARSHA, KIDDUSHIN 2b

In order to accommodate and support the developing fetus, the body undergoes significant changes. There are specific anatomical adjustments which are characteristic to certain stages of pregnancy, but each woman responds to pregnancy in her own unique way. Subsequently, even for the same mother, no two pregnancies are alike.

This chapter discusses the various body changes and why they happen, as well as offering positive suggestions for feeling good during pregnancy.

Morning Sickness

Although it can happen any time during the day or evening, nausea during pregnancy is usually referred to as "morning sickness." For many women, nausea is part and parcel of being pregnant, with most women experiencing morning sickness primarily during the first three months. Some women have only a mild sensation of nausea, while others actually vomit. Then again, some women have all the luck and never feel any discomfort.

The exact cause of nausea during pregnancy is unknown. Increased amounts of hormones such as estrogen and hCG are contributing factors, and the drastic fluctuations in blood sugar levels which occur throughout the day, especially in the early morning, also influence the way you feel.

What can you do to relieve the nausea? First of all, make sure you are eating properly. A pregnant woman should never allow her stomach to be completely empty. If you wake up in the middle of the night, take a light snack of crackers, yogurt or fruit. When you wake up in the morning, eat something light as soon as possible. Small, frequent meals which are high in carbohydrates and vitamin B6 (e.g., bananas, leafy greens, wheat germ, whole grains and wheat) have been reported to help prevent nausea. *American Health* magazine published the results of a recent (1992) study conducted at the University of Iowa, in which vitamin B6 was shown to reduce vomiting and ease nausea symptoms. However, women are cautioned against taking large doses (above the R.D.A. of 2.2 mg.) without medical supervision. Greasy foods, which are often the cause of digestive discomfort, should be avoided.

Eating at least one hour before starting out on a trip is advisable. Sitting at the front of the bus or car will help ease motion sickness. (Carrying a plastic bag, just in case, is a good idea.) Always have sucking candies or crackers handy for low-glucose episodes.

The doctor should be consulted if you begin to feel very weak or vomit excessively. Nausea usually tapers off by the 12th to 16th week of pregnancy, and with time you will be feeling better.

Heartburn and Constipation   During pregnancy, the pressure of the growing uterus on the stomach and the shift of the intestines to the side tend to slow digestive activity and can cause heartburn and constipation.

HEARTBURN is a burning sensation along the esophagus and in the stomach. It is most intense in the third trimester, when the fundus of the uterus is at its highest level.

There are several simple remedies which may help relieve heartburn: eating smaller and more frequent meals; eating almonds; not lying down immediately after eating; drinking a glass of cold water or milk. If none of these bring relief, your doctor may prescribe an antacid which is compatible with pregnancy.

CONSTIPATION is another common complaint among pregnant women. In addition to the influence of intestinal shifting and elevated hormone production, constipation can also be brought on by certain iron supplements.

See Chapter 8 on Nutrition for a more detailed discussion on preventing constipation. The rule of thumb is to increase your intake of fruits, vegetables and fluids, and get enough exercise to stimulate bowel activity. These actions will usually allay digestive disturbances.

Urinary Tract Problems

Frequent urination can literally keep a pregnant woman running day and night. During the first three months of pregnancy, before the uterus rises above the pelvis, it presses against the bladder. Pressure on the bladder may return toward the end of pregnancy, again causing frequent urination.

Although frequent urination is considered normal in pregnancy, when accompanied by burning or pain in the stomach or back, the urine needs to be tested to rule out a urinary tract infection. Pregnant women are prone to urinary tract infections because the enlarged uterus tends to obstruct the ureters, preventing sufficient emptying of the bladder. Hormonal changes during pregnancy also influence the smooth muscle tone of the urinary tract, causing the inefficient passage of urine. Urinary tract infections should be treated promptly to prevent pyelonephritis (kidney infection), which requires hospitalization and antibiotics administered intravenously.

Circulatory Changes

Circulating blood volume increases as much as 30-50% during pregnancy.[1] The circulatory system, the heart and veins in particular, must therefore assume an extra workload.

Varicose Veins   Varicose veins (varicosities) are a result of strain on the blood vessels. In response to the pressures of a heavy uterus and additional blood volume, veins are forced to exert extra effort to pump the blood back to the heart. The tiny valves responsible for pumping may falter under pressure, causing a pooling of blood. The veins then become engorged, inflamed and painful.

Varicosities may appear in the legs, the pelvic area and rectum. Varicose veins in the legs do not usually occur until after the first pregnancy, and then increase with each succeeding pregnancy. The incidence of varicose veins is strongly influenced by heredity. Thus, if your mother had varicosities, the probability is higher that you, too, will develop them.

Those who suffer from varicose veins in the legs can lessen the degree of their discomfort by taking at least two rest periods a day with feet elevated. Elevation of the feet facilitates the return of venous blood to the heart. Therefore, it is helpful to sleep with a couple of phone books or pillows under the foot of the mattress to elevate your legs. Exercise can also stimulate venous return.

You may also need to wear support hose or elastic stockings. Different types of support hose are recommended depending upon the severity of the varicosities. To prevent the pooling of blood in the legs, put on the stockings before getting out of bed in the morning; also, lie down with your feet elevated for at least five minutes before putting on support stockings after bathing or showering.

Warning! Avoid wearing knee-high stockings which can constrict venous return on a regular basis. Cotton knee-highs are a good substitute.

Symptoms such as swelling, tenderness, pain, and warmth over the calf area are symptomatic of thrombophlebitis, which requires immediate medical attention.

HEMORRHOIDS are varicosities of the rectal veins. Both heredity and constipation problems contribute to the development of hemorrhoids.

Taking a warm bath is a natural, relaxing way to alleviate hemorrhoidal symptoms. Two 20-minute baths daily in warm, soapy water for five days will bring welcome relief to an acute attack of hemorrhoids.

Another treatment to prevent hemorrhoids or relieve the pressure on existing ones, is to rest in a knee-to-chest position with hips high in the air, twice a day. This might cause a light-headed feeling at first, but gradually the pregnant woman will build up her endurance and be able to hold the position for fifteen minutes at a time.

These treatments also work to relieve varicosities in the pelvic area, which can cause pain when walking and during intimate relations. Additional relief can be achieved by wearing support hose with a thick sanitary napkin.

Heart Palpitations

Another possible side effect of increased circulating blood volume is heart palpitations. These are not a cause for worry — the pounding sensations are quite normal. Palpitations will occur less frequently if you avoid sudden movements and change positions slowly. Discuss these symptoms with your doctor, as dormant heart problems are sometimes detected during pregnancy.

Blood Pressure

Blood pressure is measured using a fractionate number. The upper number measures systolic pressure, and the lower number diastolic. Average blood pressure varies, but is usually about 120/70 mmHg in women of childbearing age.

HYPOTENSION

It is common for blood pressure to drop during pregnancy, and 90/60 is still considered normal. Symptoms of low blood pressure include dizziness, fatigue and feeling faint. To overcome these symptoms, simply increase your fluid intake.

Two forms of low blood pressure — supine hypotension and orthostatic hypotension can be easily prevented without medical intervention.

SUPINE HYPOTENSION is caused by lying flat on your back. The enlarged uterus depresses the inferior vena cava, reducing the efficiency of blood circulation. When this happens, you may become pale, feel faint and experience a racing heartbeat. It is, therefore, advisable to avoid lying on your back for more than four minutes at a time when pregnant. Lying on your left side is the best position, as it maximizes both blood circulation throughout the body and blood flow to your baby.

Anyone, pregnant or not, can experience ORTHOSTATIC HYPOTENSION. Rising quickly from a lying position can cause dizziness, so get up slowly. Sit first and then stand.

HYPERTENSION

High blood pressure in pregnancy is a dangerous and potentially life-threatening condition. When a woman begins her pregnancy with high blood pressure, "chronic hypertension" is noted in her medical record. She should receive special prenatal care and often continues taking the same medication during pregnancy that she took before pregnancy.

PREGNANCY-INDUCED HYPERTENSION develops after the 20th week of pregnancy. Symptoms include excess swelling in the hands, face, feet and legs. It is hard to open and close the hands, protein is detected in the urine, and there is a sudden increase in body weight. Blurring of vision and flashes of light accompanied by a headache should be considered serious warning signs of high blood pressure. However, it is the actual rise in blood pressure that is the most significant symptom of high blood pressure.

Systolic pressure can fluctuate from one minute to the next in response to nerves or pain. Diastolic pressure is the more prominent indicator of hypertension. The rise of diastolic pressure in a pregnant woman above the normal range of 60 or 70 to 90 mmHg can be a sign of trouble. If resting at home does not lower the elevated blood pressure, hospitalization with medication and strict bed rest is required.

Severe high blood pressure in pregnancy (diastolic pressure above 90) is called TOXEMIA or PRE-ECLAMPSIA It can lead to maternal convulsions (eclampsia) which are harmful to both mother and fetus. In order to prevent further harm to the mother or baby, toxemia which cannot be controlled by bed rest and medication requires the termination of pregnancy — the early delivery of the baby, usually by cesarean section.

As the pregnancy advances and the fetus grows heavier, the pressure on muscles, ligaments and bones affects the general structure of your body. As a result, the most common complaints are back pain and muscle tension. Rest and exercise are both helpful in relieving back strain, and a warm shower or bubble bath can relax muscle tension.

Muscular-Skeletal Changes

Most of the burden of carrying the "expanded you" falls on your feet, legs, and back, so make life more comfortable by wearing shoes that fit and avoid high heels. Don't be surprised if you find that you need wider, larger shoes while you are pregnant. As a matter of fact, your shoe size may never return to what it was before, as these changes might persist even after you have given birth.

In addition to the aforementioned minor discomforts, there are several specific conditions which are attributed to muscular-skeletal changes in pregnancy: leg cramps, round ligament pain and sciatic pain.

LEG CRAMPS: usually occur during sleep or upon awakening in the morning. The first time you experience a leg cramp you may be quite surprised by the extreme pain, the intensity of which can even be compared to labor. The calf muscle will become as hard as a rock. To release the cramp, straighten your leg and flex your toes upward. Your husband can help by flexing your foot and forcefully massaging your calf. Standing on the affected leg will bring immediate relief.

To prevent leg cramps, avoid pointing your toes in bed and increase your dietary intake of calcium. Taking a prescribed calcium supplement will often preclude frequent recurrence of leg cramps.

ROUND LIGAMENT PAIN: Often pregnancy will cause pressure on the round ligaments which support the uterus, resulting in a sharp, pulling pain on either side of the lower abdomen. This uncomfortable — and sometimes frightening — sensation is aggravated by rising too quickly from a prone position. The recommended method of rising is to turn from your side to a sitting position, and only then stand up. Massage and heat applications are also helpful.

SCIATIC PAIN: The fetus may assume a position which specifically puts pressure on the sciatic nerve. This may cause sharp, shooting pain across the lower back and down the legs. Changing your position and applying heat may provide temporary relief.

Hormonal   Hormones are the biggest scapegoats in pregnancy.
Changes   Hormonal changes can be blamed for everything, from mood swings to the way you look and feel.

PROGESTERONE is called the "pregnancy hormone." It serves to maintain the uterine lining, support the function of the placenta, and prevent premature contractions. During the first trimester of pregnancy, the sudden increase of progesterone (along with other hormones) causes extraordinary fatigue. This hormonal shift is also responsible for the reduction in sexual drive (libido). This is only a temporary "down," and you will usually experience a resurgence of strength by the fourth month of pregnancy.

ESTROGEN contributes to mammary gland development in preparation for lactation, and stimulates the uterus to expand with the developing fetus. At first the ovaries produce the extra estrogen, but afterwards the placenta takes over this task. The amount of estrogen in the blood (estriol) is often tested to evaluate the condition of the pregnancy.

Increased estrogen levels can cause the following symptoms:

Stuffy Nose and Nosebleeds — During pregnancy, some women have a persistent stuffy nose, which is neither an allergy nor a cold. It disappears after delivery. It is best to blow your nose gently to avoid nosebleeds, which are also common during pregnancy. Frequent or heavy nosebleeds should be reported to the doctor.

Dental Problems — Increased estrogen in the system can cause puffy gums, which are prone to bleeding and can become a chronic condition. Take meticulous care of teeth and gums during pregnancy, and have regular dental check-ups and cleanings to avoid gum problems.

Vascular Spiders — Small broken capillaries may appear on the legs, and palms may become unusually red. These symptoms need not alarm you, as they are natural consequences of the increased estrogen level during pregnancy.

Vaginal Discharge — Many women experience a white, watery vaginal discharge during pregnancy. In addition to the high estrogen level, the increased blood supply to the vagina and cervix contribute to this discharge. To prevent discomfort and potential infection (especially yeast infection [monilia]), wear loose clothing. Cotton underwear is a must. Any discomfort or increased discharge should be reported to your doctor.

Anticipating Menstruation (Onah)

The most significant hormonal change in pregnancy is the cessation of menstruation. During the first three months of pregnancy the laws of *niddah* apply as usual. This means that if a woman had a *veses kavua* (a set pattern for the date of her menstruation), for the first three months she must separate from her husband on her anticipation date. If she had a *veses she'eino kavua* (an irregular pattern for the date of her menstruation), the laws of separation apply only for the first month.[2] These laws must be observed even if she knows without a doubt that she is pregnant.[3]

After the first three months of pregnancy, a woman

may disregard her fixed anticipation date, and the regular laws of separation no longer apply.

If a woman sees blood even after the first three months of pregnancy, she must observe the laws of *taharah* (family purity) as prescribed. She must also separate the next month on her anticipation date (following the laws of a *veses she'eino kavua*). Even if she were to see blood on three consecutive dates (which would normally put her in the category of having a *veses kavua*), she is only required to anticipate the next *onah* according to the laws of a *veses she'eino kavua*.[4] Consult your Rav for clarification.

Skin Changes   During pregnancy, the pituitary gland becomes enlarged, causing noticeable skin color changes. Pigmentation changes vary with each woman according to her skin shade and complexion. The skin usually returns to its normal color after delivery.

A dark brown line may develop from the navel to the pubic bone. This dark streak is called the "linea nigra" and will fade after delivery. Also, some women temporarily develop a "mask of pregnancy" (chloasma), brown streaks on their cheeks and across the nose.

Stretch marks (striae gravidarum) can appear on the abdomen, buttocks, thighs and breasts. These brownish-red lines are caused by the stretching and breakdown of the elastic fibers of the skin. The color lasts only through pregnancy, fading to a silvery shade after delivery, when hormones return to their normal level.

Although skin changes may be unavoidable during pregnancy, it is important to keep the skin supple and moisturized. It is not recommended to overexpose yourself to the sun, and if you are in the sun even for a very short time, you should use sunscreen on your face.

Diabetes in Pregnancy   Insulin is a hormone which facilitates the transformation of glucose into energy. It is necessary for the pancreas to increase insulin production during pregnancy to meet the greater demand for energy.

Women who do not produce enough insulin to respond to the higher demands of pregnancy (approximately 2-3% of pregnant women) suffer from gestational diabetes. Gestational diabetes usually disappears after pregnancy, but 50-60% of this group will develop maturity-onset diabetes (type II) ten to fifteen years later.[5]

Elevated glucose levels may be detected through routine urine or blood tests. All women with a family history of diabetes should undergo additional blood testing at the beginning of their third trimester.

Gestational diabetes may be controlled by following a carefully designed meal plan. Some women may need daily insulin injections in addition to a strict diet to maintain the proper glucose-insulin balance. Women who are diabetic receive special obstetrical care to ensure a successful outcome.

Diabetes in pregnancy can be very dangerous. The acidotic result of a glucose-insulin imbalance can be toxic to the fetus. Placental function also decreases dramatically at the end of a diabetic pregnancy, limiting the amount of oxygen and nutrients available to the fetus. Moreover, the over-stimulation of the pituitary growth hormone causes a larger-sized fetus, which may cause difficulties in normal delivery.

The newborn himself may suffer from hypoglycemia as he no longer receives the glucose-enriched diet from his diabetic mother. His own glucose-insulin balance will need to be strictly monitored. Therefore, a pregnant woman with diabetes can expect to be hospitalized sometime between the 36th and 38th week of pregnancy, and labor is usually induced by the 38th week. The cesarean rate is significantly higher in diabetic mothers.

Humble Appreciation

In relating the story of the birth of Yitzchak, the Torah says: "And Hashem remembered Sarah as *He had said* and Hashem did unto Sarah as *He had spoken.*"[6]

Why did the Torah say "as He had said" and "as He

had spoken," when either one would have sufficed? What do these extra words teach us?

Rashi explains that "as He had said" refers to her pregnancy, and "as He had spoken" refers to the birth.[7] Yet this does not fully answer the question. For if God fulfilled His promise regarding the birth, surely a pregnancy must precede it. If so, why would there be a separate mention of pregnancy? Why did God promise Sarah both a birth and a pregnancy?

As much as women look forward to cradling a newborn in their arms, they do not look forward to the pregnancy. Wouldn't it be nice if we could just give birth without the aches and pains, morning sickness, leg cramps, weight gain, back problems, and all the other side effects of pregnancy?

However, with all its discomforts, pregnancy is not only a means to an end, but also a blessing in itself. Sarah certainly thought so. She did not only desire a son, but she also yearned for the experience of being pregnant.

Perhaps the reason is that there is something very feminine about a pregnant woman. Sarah was barren, but she did not merely have a fertility problem — she actually did not have a uterus.[8] Therefore, Sarah truly wished she could become pregnant. And when Hashem remembered her, He remembered how important the pregnancy was to her. For this reason, He placed special mention of the pregnancy in the Torah. God remembered what "He had said" — that she would be pregnant — and what "He had spoken" — she would give birth.

The same desire for pregnancy was shared by Rivkah as well. For Rivkah referred to her unusual pregnancy, saying, "*Lamah zeh anochi* — Why is this for me?"[9] Rashi interprets this as, "Why did I crave to be pregnant?" Rashi's use of the term "pregnant" as opposed to "have children" implies that Rivkah also had a special desire to be pregnant.

The hardships of pregnancy are dwarfed in comparison with the way a woman feels about the opportunity to fulfill her femininity.

Rivkah experienced an especially difficult pregnancy and therefore went to "inquire of Hashem." Rashi says that she went to the *beis midrash* of Shem to find out what would be the outcome of the pregnancy. Rabbi Avraham Bakrat in his commentary notes that Rivkah's concern and prayers were to know what would come of this peculiar pregnancy, but she did not pray to Hashem to ease her pains.[10]

We take for granted so much of the bounty which God showers upon us. A woman with fertility problems would give up everything for the privilege of becoming pregnant, with all it entails. As Rachel said to Ya'akov, "Give me children or I will die."[11] Expectant mothers are very fortunate. Not everyone merits this blessing. It requires our most humble appreciation.

NOTES

1. J.A. Pritchard, P.C. MacDonald, eds., *Williams Obstetrics*, 17th ed. (New York: Appleton-Century Croft, 1985).
2. *Yoreh De'ah* 189:33. However, she still anticipates her *onah beinonis* on the 60th and 90th day from her last period (*Darkei Taharah*, p. 84).
3. R. Akiva Eiger, *Responsa*, ch. 128; R. Moshe Feinstein, *Responsa* published in R. Shimon Eider, *Hilchos Niddah*.
4. *Yoreh De'ah* 189:33.
5. J. Folkman, H. J. Hollerorth, *A Guide for Women with Diabetes Who Are Pregnant... Or Plan to Be* (Boston: Joslin Diabetes Center, 1986), p. 8.
6. *Bereshis* 21:1.
7. Ibid., Rashi.
8. *Yevamos* 64a.
9. *Bereshis* 25:22.
10. R. Avraham Bakrat, *Sefer Ha-Zikaron*, 15th-century commentary on Rashi.
11. *Bereshis* 30:2.

6 | Safe Pregnancy Guidelines

The greatest of fortunes is good health.

BEN SIRA 30, 16

Every pregnant woman is concerned about taking the proper precautions to insure the birth of a healthy baby. Therefore she should also avoid certain environmental agents which can harm the developing fetus.

A teratogen is a toxin which has the ability to penetrate the placenta and damage the developing fetus, resulting in birth defects or even spontaneous abortion. The fetus is most vulnerable to teratogens during the first three months of pregnancy when the internal organs and limbs are being formed. During the second and third trimesters, toxins may inhibit both structural and neurological growth. Thus, in addition to physical disabilities, exposure to toxins can cause behavioral problems.

Unfortunately many destructive agents pervade our environment. Although it is impossible to avoid all exposure, an effort must be made to keep such exposure to a minimum. The following is a discussion of the most common dangers to which a pregnant woman may be exposed.

Tobacco   We have all been educated about the hazards of smoking. Even the Chafetz Chayim, who lived at the turn of this century, was aware of the dangers of cigarette smoking.[1]

A pregnant woman who smokes reduces the probability of a favorable outcome to her pregnancy.[2] Smoking acts as a lethal teratogen which, in addition to causing low birth weight (a decrease of 7 oz. or more),[3] has
also been associated with increased spontaneous abortions and placental abnormalities.[4]

Cigarette smoke robs the fetus of oxygen and nutrients which are required for growth. Fetal heart rates recorded while the mother smokes are elevated, indicating
fetal distress. Even passive smoking — breathing smoke
from the atmosphere when someone else has been
smoking — adversely affects the fetus, the newborn, and
anyone else in the vicinity. It is, therefore, wise to avoid
a smoky environment at all times.

Alcohol

Fetal alcohol syndrome (FAS) is the name of the
collection of irreversible consequences of alcohol
consumption during pregnancy. The abnormalities characteristic of FAS include growth retardation, mental retardation, abnormal development of various body organs
and facial abnormalities.

Even light drinking — as little as two drinks a week
— can handicap the fetus. Since we do not know if there
is a minimum amount of liquor which is safe during
pregnancy, the best precaution is to avoid alcohol consumption altogether.[5] (Of course, a small sip of wine at
Kiddush would not be a problem.)

Caffeine

According to the United States Food and Drug Administration, "prudence dictates that pregnant women avoid
caffeine-containing products or use them sparingly."[6]

Many studies document the effects of caffeine consumption during pregnancy. The common consensus is
that caffeine intake should be limited to no more than
300 mg. per day. Caffeine intake above this maximum
allowance is known to decrease infant birth weight.[7]

The consumption of even moderate amounts of caffeine (151 mg. or more daily) has been linked to spontaneous abortions.[8] However, at this time there is no direct

evidence of caffeine use being associated with fetal growth retardation (impaired growth while in utero) or malformations.[9]

Taking into consideration the fact that caffeine enters breast milk, another study advises the nursing mother to consume less than a moderate level.[10] Caffeine intake while nursing may be linked to colic and infant sleeplessness.

The following is a list of approximate caffeine values, which vary according to the caffeine strength of the individual product:

coffee (brewed)	100-150 mg. per cup
coffee (instant)	60-80 mg. per cup
tea	40-100 mg. per cup
cola	32-65 mg./11 oz. (340 ml.)
chocolate	21.2 mg/3.5 oz. bar
cocoa	5-10 mg. per serving[11]

Drugs   The use of any addictive drug is harmful to both mother and fetus. Women during their childbearing years should be aware that drug abuse also interferes with fertility.

Initial studies of cocaine use during pregnancy indicate that in addition to severe birth defects, cocaine use may even cause sudden fetal death.[12] Babies born to drug-addicted mothers are themselves addicted. These newborn infants display severe withdrawal symptoms requiring intense medical treatment, including sedation. Many of these newborns do not even survive.

Drugs such as marijuana, cocaine and heroin also pass into breast milk and affect the nursing baby.

Medication   The expectant mother must fully understand that all medications, whether prescription or over-the-counter, become a part of the maternal blood stream and are transferred through the placenta to the fetus. Under certain circumstances, even medication prescribed by a physician can harm the fetus. Many lice shampoos and hair dyes are not recommended for use during pregnancy and nursing.

Although many drugs have been proven safe for use during pregnancy, it is best to avoid taking any unnecessary medication. Before taking any drug, even medicine prescribed by a dentist or another doctor, the obstetrician should be consulted to make sure it is safe to use during pregnancy. Acetaminophen (Tylenol/Acamol) is considered safe for use during pregnancy and lactation.[13]

Infectious Diseases

Rubella (German measles) can cause a great deal of damage to the developing fetus. It is the most commonly feared, yet the most preventable illness that a pregnant woman can incur. Most women have been vaccinated against rubella during childhood and adolescence. Those who have not been vaccinated, should use the opportunity right after birth to get immunization.

Generally speaking, any fever over 101°F, or 38.5°C, should be treated by a doctor. Acetaminophen, not aspirin, is recommended to bring down fever and relieve aches and pains.

Radiation

Although exposure to high doses of radiation or unnecessary diagnostic x-rays should be avoided during pregnancy, in certain instances it may be medically preferable for a woman to undergo an x-ray procedure. According to an article published by the Israel Medical Association, there is no danger to the fetus from the minimal amount of radiation in dental x-rays or even a head x-ray. Thus, proper dental care or pertinent diagnostic examinations can be carried out during pregnancy. The obstetrician can determine the necessity and safety of any potential procedure. The pelvic area should be covered by a protective lead apron when exposed to radiation, whether or not a woman is pregnant.[14]

Environmental Pollutants and Toxins

In order to avoid all environmental hazards, we would have to live in a sterile bubble. Many pollutants in the air, food, and water are unavoidable. However, the expectant mother should make every effort to bypass areas of dense pollution and insure that her food and water are as toxin-free as possible.

Some pregnant women are exposed to chemical toxins, toxic wastes, or radiation at work. A woman who suspects that these toxic agents exist in her work environment should consult her employers and her local environmental protection agency. It is a woman's responsibility to get the appropriate information regarding potential harm to the fetus or threats to her fertility.

Travel Although pregnancy is not considered an illness, special attention should be given to travel arrangements while pregnant.

Traveling by plane is not considered problematic before the 32nd week of pregnancy. Many airlines require a doctor's note if a woman wishes to fly after this time. A well-pressurized cabin (as is found in commercial aircraft) makes jet travel safe for a healthy pregnant woman. She should ask for a seat in the nonsmoking section and avoid sitting for extended periods. Drinking plenty of fluids is a must as plane travel can be very dehydrating.

When traveling long distances by car, plan brief stops for stretching and exercise to promote circulation. Seatbelts should be positioned low across the lap — not across the uterus. Though some localities may be lax about requiring a pregnant woman to wear a seat belt, seat belts can save the lives of both mother and baby, when worn properly.

Protecting Your Health We are commanded not to unnecessarily destroy any of Hashem's creations. For example, the Torah explicitly states, "When you lay siege to a city and wage war against it a long time to capture it, you must not destroy its trees, wielding an ax against them; for you may eat of them..."[15]

The prohibition against wanton destruction applies to property as well as to nature. Causing damage to or destroying one's clothes or utensils is also considered a transgression of this commandment.[16]

Although we are most familiar with this prohibition in reference to wasting food, its most serious violation is represented by one who endangers his own body. The Talmud tells us that, "One who gave blood and became chilled may break furniture to use for firewood if no firewood is available." When Abaye objects and calls this wanton destruction, his teacher, Rabbah, answers that despite the fact that it is wanton destruction, endangering one's body is a far more serious crime.[17]

Rabbenu Yonah concludes in *Sha'arei Teshuvah*: "We were warned not to destroy our body by endangering it."[18] And while the Rambam does not rule that one who abuses his health violates the prohibition against wanton destruction, he does say that proper care of one's health is considered emulating the ways of Hashem.[19]

There are different degrees of endangering one's health. Obviously one cannot compare drinking too much coffee to the gravity of serious drug abuse. Different health hazards lead to varying consequences, and the *halachah* is determined accordingly. Our Rabbis strongly advise against consuming that which is harmful to us, yet they do not necessarily forbid it.[20] Willful exposure to serious health hazards, on the other hand, is actually considered a transgression against Torah law.[21]

Whether there is an *issur d'Oraysa* (prohibition stipulated by the Torah) or not, *Chazal's* advice for avoiding danger and harm carries a clear message. The Be'er Ha-Golah expresses this message succinctly at the end of his commentary on the *Shulchan Aruch*: "One who endangers himself behaves as if he is displeased with the will of his Creator. He doesn't want to serve Him nor does he covet His reward. There can be no greater disregard of Hashem's Law or display of irreverence."[22]

And in that spirit the Rambam advised his son: "It should be known that a healthy body precedes a healthy soul. And this is the key to the gates of Heaven."[23]

NOTES

1. *Zechor L'Miryam*, ch. 23; *see also Iggros Moshe, Choshen Mishpat*, vol. II, 76.
2. N. Hacker, J. Moore, *Essentials of Obstetrics and Gynecology* (Philadelphia: W.B. Saunders Company, 1986), p. 77.
3. L. Holmes, P. Pober, and M. Werler, *Teratogen Update — Environmentally Induced Birth Defect Risks* (New York: Alan R. Liss, Inc., 1986) pp. 131-39.
4. E. Lanmer, A. Mitchell, L. Rosenberg, M. Werler, "Maternal Cigarette Smoking during Pregnancy," *American Journal of Epidemiology*, 132(5):926, (Johns Hopkins University, 1990).
5. J. Kline, P. Shrout, Z. Stein, et al.: "Drinking During Pregnancy and Spontaneous Abortion," *Lancet* 1:176, 1980.
6. "Caffeine and Pregnancy," *U.S. Food and Drug Administration Bulletin* 10:19, 1980.
7. C.J. Hogue, "Coffee in Pregnancy," *Lancet* 1:554, 1981.
8. W.D. Todd, D.F. Tapley, eds., *Columbia University Complete Guide to Pregnancy* (New York: Crown Publishers, 1988), p. 107.
9. M. Evans, C. Lin, *Intrauterine Growth Retardation* (New York: McGraw-Hill, 1984), p. 136.
10. A. Berger, "Effects of Caffeine Consumption on Pregnancy Outcome," *Journal of Reproductive Medicine*, 33(11):945, 1988.
11. Ibid.; *see also* C. Flinders, L. Robertson, B. Ruppenthal, *Laurel's Kitchen* (Berkeley: Ten Speed Press, 1986), p. 373.
12. O.P. Heinonen, S. Shapiro, D. Stone, *Birth Defects and Drugs in Pregnancy* (Littleton Co., Publishing Sciences Group, 1977).
13. A. Evans, K. Niswander, *Manual of Obstetrics* (Boston: Little, Brown & Co., 1991), p. 29.
14. J. Arnon, A. Ornoy, "Teratological Counseling in Israel," *HaRefuah — Journal of the Israel Medical Association* 120:10 (May 1991).
15. *Devarim* 20:19.
16. Rambam, *Hilchos Avelus* 14: 23, 24.
17. *Shabbos* 129a.
18. *Sha'arei Teshuvah*, Gate Three, ch. 82.
19. Rambam, *Hilchos De'os* 4:1; *see also* R. Menachem Slae, *Smoking and Damage to Health in the Halachah* (Jerusalem: Feldheim Publishers).
20. Ibid.; *see also, Shulchan Aruch, Choshen Mishpat* 427; *Iggros Moshe, Choshen Mishpat*, vol. II, 76.
21. *See Aruch Ha-Shulchan, Choshen Mishpat* 427:8.
22. Be'er Ha-Golah, *Choshen Mishpat* 427.
23. *See* Hebrew appendix.

7 | Fasting during Pregnancy

*And you should keep My statutes and My
ordinances, which if a man does, he shall
live by them; I am the Lord.*

VAYIKRA 18:5

The Torah instructs us to fast on Yom Kippur, as it **Yom Kippur**
is written (*Vayikra 23:27*), *"V'inisem es naf-
shoseichem* — You shall afflict your souls." The Rabbis
explain this to mean that we should refrain from eating
and drinking.

The obligation to fast on Yom Kippur usually applies
to pregnant women as well.[1] A healthy woman who does
not anticipate any problems during pregnancy is usually
able to fulfill this requirement without too much difficulty. However, there are pregnant women with medical
problems who are not allowed to fast on Yom Kippur,
lest fasting induce complications which may prove dangerous for mother and baby.

It is crucial to accept the fact that a pregnant woman
who is given a *heter* (Rabbinic permission) to eat on Yom
Kippur must eat; she is not allowed to fast. Her mitzvah
is to follow the advice of her doctor and Rav to eat and
drink. The problem is that psychologically it is much
easier to fulfill the mitzvah of fasting than the "mitzvah
of eating," especially when one understands the significance of Yom Kippur and feels strange having to eat on a

day when everyone else is fasting. One must realize, however, that just as Hashem told us to fast on Yom Kippur, He also told us to listen to our doctors and rabbis when they tell us to eat if fasting is considered dangerous. In this regard, it is written (*Koheles* 7:16), "*Al tiheyeh tzaddik harbeh* — Don't be overly righteous." And the Torah says (*Vayikra* 18:5), "*V'chai bahem* — Live by them." The statutes of the Torah are to be observed without endangering our lives.[2]

A woman who falls into the categories described below should consult both with her doctor and her Rav to determine if her personal situation allows her to fast:

❧ In the case of medical problems such as high blood pressure or diabetes, a woman may be told not to fast, and her Rav must also tell her if she should eat only measured portions (*shiurim* — see glossary). In certain circumstances she will be told to drink but not eat; sometimes both eating and drinking are permitted, with or without *shiurim*. Every woman and every pregnancy is evaluated according to different criteria.

❧ If a woman is told by her doctor that fasting can cause premature labor, or if she has a history of miscarriages or premature deliveries, then the ruling generally is that she should eat according to *shiurim*.[3]

❧ When a pregnant woman with no specific medical problems tries to fast and experiences extreme weakness to the point that she is unable to get out of bed, a doctor should be asked if she must eat. If a doctor is not available, her family must see to it that she eats, even if she claims it is not necessary, because she has the status of an ill person in danger and is obligated to eat.[4]

❧ A pregnant woman who faints or feels close to fainting should be fed until she recovers her equilibrium.[5]

❧ A woman who began experiencing contractions before the 37th week of pregnancy should drink sweet water or juice without *shiurim*.[6] During the sixth, seventh and eighth months of pregnancy (weeks 28-36), the

expectant mother is especially vulnerable to fluid deprivation. Dehydration can cause premature contractions
and even cervical dilation. If contractions do not stop after an hour, she should seek medical attention.

❧ A woman who is very ill (even if she is not in immediate danger but her not taking medication may lead
to a dangerous illness), or a woman who is on medication for a chronic condition, should consult her doctor
and Rav about taking pills or syrup on Yom Kippur.
Some authorities allow swallowing pills or syrup without
water for serious illnesses. If the woman is unable to
take the medication without water, she may sip a little
water with the pill.[7]

❧ If a woman smells and craves a certain food and
asks for it, or if it is obvious from the expression on her
face that she needs it, she may be allowed to eat that
food in portions which are less than a *shiur* until she
feels better.[8]

❧ Every woman would like to go to shul on Yom Kippur. However, it is better to stay at home and rest and
continue fasting than to go to shul and then become so
weak that one is forced to eat.[9]

More details about Yom Kippur and eating with *shiurim* can be found in Chapter 17, p. 193.

The Seventeenth of Tammuz, The Fast of Gedalyah,   **Minor Fast**
The Tenth of Teves, and The Fast of Esther are mi-   **Days**
nor fast days instituted by the Rabbis. The following rules apply to pregnant women with respect to the
minor fast days:

❧ A pregnant woman is exempt from fasting after the
fortieth day of pregnancy (54 days from the previous
menstruation). Before the fortieth day, a woman is obligated to fast unless she feels very weak, nauseous or
suffers much discomfort.[10]

❧ If a pregnant woman feels weak or has discomfort,
she should not fast. This holds true even if it can be de-

termined that fasting will not endanger the fetus.[11]

❧ A strong woman who fasts easily and experiences no discomfort may fast if she so desires.[12]

❧ When a pregnant woman does not fast on a minor fast day, she does not have to make it up another time.[13]

Tisha B'Av Although the fast of Tisha B'Av (the Ninth of Av) was instituted by the Rabbis (d'Rabbanan), which normally would exempt a pregnant woman, commemorating the sadness of the day is so important that everyone is obligated to fast, even pregnant women.[14] Nevertheless, under certain circumstances a pregnant woman may be exempt from fasting.

❧ On Tisha B'Av, there are different considerations for granting permission to eat than on Yom Kippur. On Yom Kippur, we must first determine whether or not it is dangerous to fast. But on Tisha B'Av, illness, or the possibility that not eating will cause illness, permits a person to eat, even if he or she is not in danger.[15] Many poskim in Israel are flexible in this regard, for they take into account the intense heat of summer in the Middle East and the fact that nowadays people are generally weaker (yardah chulshah l'olam). Therefore any pregnant woman who feels that she cannot fast, lest it lead to illness or extreme weakness, should consult her Rav.[16]

❧ If her doctor suspects that fasting might cause premature contractions, the woman should not fast.[17]

❧ A woman who is under treatment for high blood pressure or diabetes or needs to stay in bed, or a woman with any other complication in pregnancy is not obligated to fast, for Chazal did not require that the sick fast on Tisha B'Av.[18]

Other conditions which permit a woman to eat on Tisha B'Av are anemia, low blood pressure, dizziness, pressure in the abdominal area related to pregnancy, heart palpitations, fever, or any unusual pain which can be caused by the pregnancy or any illness.

Some authorities say that a woman who is allowed to eat on Tisha B'Av may eat right away, without any waiting at all. However, according to some opinions, a woman who is allowed to eat on Tisha B'Av should try to fast for a few hours, but if this is difficult, she may eat immediately.[19]

A Rav needs to be consulted to determine if a woman who is allowed to eat on Tisha B'Av must eat according to shiurim, as is the case on Yom Kippur. Some opinions suggest that, if possible, she should eat less than a shiur in order to maintain the status of fasting. However, some say that no shiurim are applicable on Tisha B'Av, since Tisha B'Av was instituted by the Rabbis.[20] Also, the type of illness may determine the decision.[21]

❧ A healthy woman who has a headache or does not feel well may take medicine (pills or liquid).[22] If liquid is needed in order to swallow the pill, she may take a sip of water.[23]

❧ If Tisha B'Av falls on Shabbos and the fast is deferred until Sunday, a Rav should be consulted about fasting. Some authorities say that a pregnant or nursing woman (even one who is healthy) is not required to fast.[24]

When the fast of Tisha B'Av is deferred until Sunday, a woman who is allowed to eat should make Havdalah (without the spices) before she eats. However, if she does not eat until morning, she should also wait to say Havdalah until the morning.[25]

More details concerning Tisha B'Av can be found in Chapter 17, p. 194.

❧ A pregnant woman who is allowed to eat and drink should only eat what is necessary to sustain her.[26] Although pregnancy exempts a woman from fasting on minor fast days and medical complications exempt her from fasting on Tisha B'Av, she is still obligated to feel sadness because of the destruction of the Temple. We hope that with the coming of the Mashiach, these days will soon become days of joy and gladness for our people.

The Pre-Fast Meal There has been almost no scientific information as to the effect of the Jewish fast (abstinence from water as well as food) on the body. Dr. David Blondheim of Ziv Hospital in Safed, Israel, is extending a study of a decade ago by his father, Professor Hillel Blondheim of Hadassah Hospital, Jerusalem. That study defined the effects of fasting on the blood biochemistry and viscosity of normal subjects.

The new study was aimed at determining the effect of the dietary composition of the prefast meal on the ease of fasting. In the study, normal volunteers fasted for 24 hours on three occasions, each fast preceded by a meal rich in either protein, fat, or carbohydrates. After each fast the subjects listed side effects experienced, such as nausea, headache, dizziness and faintness as well as the degrees of thirst and of hunger, and the ease of the fast compared with previous religious fasts. There were more side effects in more subjects and the subjects were more thirsty after a high protein meal than after a fatty or high carbohydrate meal.

It was therefore concluded that to promote easy fasting, the pre-fast meal (seudah mafsekes) should consist of high carbohydrate and high fat foods, and contain a minimum of protein.

In another ongoing study, the effect of fasting on the pregnant woman and her fetus is being studied by Dr. Blondheim and Dr. Nili Yanai, a gynecologist at Ha-Emek Hospital in Afulah, Israel. Conclusions cannot be drawn until the study is completed.

NOTES

1. *Orach Chayim* 617:1.
2. *Responsa*, Radbaz, vol. III, 444; *Tzitz Eliezer*, vol. x, §25, ch. 14.
3. *Toras Ha-Yoledes* 50:4; also heard from R. Chaim P. Sheinberg.
4. *Aruch Ha-Shulchan* 618:1; 554:7.

5. *Iggros Moshe, Orach Chayim,* vol. IV, 121.
6. According to the medical advice of Dr. Chaim Yaffe, head of the gynecology department, Bikur Cholim Hospital, and halachically approved by R. Chaim P. Sheinberg.
7. *Responsa, Eretz Tzvi,* 88; *Iggros Moshe, Orach Chayim,* vol. III, 91.
8. *Orach Chayim,* 617:2.
9. Heard from R. Chaim P. Sheinberg.
10. *Orach Chayim* 550:1; *Mishnah Berurah* 550:3; *Orach Chayim* 554:5; *see* Hebrew appendix.
11. *Aruch Ha-Shulchan* 550:1.
12. Ibid.; *see* Hebrew appendix.
13. *Responsa, Yechaveh Da'as,* vol. I, 33.
14. *Orach Chayim* 554:5.
15. Tur, in the name of Ramban, 554; *Aruch Ha-Shulchan* 554:7.
16. *Toras Ha-Yoledes* 48, note 8; *Responsa, Yechaveh Da'as,* vol. I, 42.
17. If he has good reason to suspect complications.
18. *Aruch Ha-Shulchan* 554:7; *see* Hebrew appendix for full quote.
19. *See* Hebrew appendix, ch. 17, note 35.
20. *See Mishnah Berurah,* 554: *biur halachah,* "*D'Ba-Makom*"; *Aruch Ha-Shulchan* 554:7, and *Tzitz Eliezer,* vol. X, §25, ch. 16.
21. *See Toras Ha-Yoledes* 48, notes 5 and 6.
22. *Tzitz Eliezer,* vol. X, §25, ch. 22.
23. Heard from R. Mordechai Eliyahu.
24. *Responsa, Yechaveh Da'as,* vol. III, 40.
25. *Kaf Ha-Chayim* 556:9.
26. *Orach Chayim* 554:5.

8 | Nutrition

A person who eats every day in order to strengthen his body to serve Hashem is as though he were fulfilling the mitzvah of eating on erev Yom Kippur, and is given reward in this world resembling Olam Ha-ba.

NEFESH KOL CHAI I, 28

To properly serve Hashem every Jew should do his utmost to guard his health. Poor health impairs one's ability to understand the Torah and fulfill its commandments.[1] Since the body is the vessel into which Hashem has entrusted the soul and the conduit for the accomplishment of spiritual goals, it is a religious obligation to maintain one's health.

We devote so much effort to supporting a spiritually rich Torah lifestyle — carefully choosing for ourselves the proper education, environment and synagogue. The strengthening and upkeep of our bodies is certainly worthy of the same conscientious attention.

A sick person is exempt from many of the mitzvos. But if the illness is due to negligent health care and reckless dietary habits, he will certainly be held accountable for his lack of effort to preserve his health, and for actively abetting the body's decline into infirmity.[2] The Talmud warns that if one is indifferent to his health care needs, *Hakadosh Baruch Hu* will likewise overlook his needs. For Hashem will then say, If he didn't take pity on his own life, why should I take pity on him?[3]

The maintenance of one's health and psychological

well-being is considered serving Hashem as much as re-fining one's *middos* or fulfilling a mitzvah. A story in the *Midrash* illustrates this dictum:

> When Hillel parted from his students, they asked him, "Rabbenu, where are you going?"
>
> Hillel replied, "I am going to fulfill a mitzvah."
>
> "Which mitzvah?" they asked.
>
> "The mitzvah of bathing."
>
> "What kind of commandment is that, to bathe?"
>
> Hillel replied: "It is certainly a mitzvah. For if attendants at museums are honorably employed and paid to wash and shine the statues, then how much more so am I, who was created in Hashem's image, obligated to take care of my body!"[4]

Many of the Sages who codified *halachah* included a chapter on proper health care in their writings. The Rambam, the *Kitzur Shulchan Aruch*, the Ben Ish Chai, the *Kaf Ha-Chayim* and the *Mishnah Berurah* all considered good health a halachic issue.

The key to good health lies mainly in our diet. Proper eating habits and the correct choice of foods will help guarantee an "illness-free" life. In fact, the National Cancer Institute has related 38% of all cancer to dietary indiscretion, making that the single most significant cause of the dreaded disease.[5]

"He who guards his mouth and his tongue will be protected from affliction," promises Shelomo *Ha-Melech*.[6] The Rambam elaborates on this teaching, explaining that "guarding one's mouth" implies eating the right foods, while "guarding one's tongue" refers to speaking properly. Combining both these warnings in one verse leads the Rambam to the conclusion that one must be just as careful of what goes into one's mouth as of what comes out of one's mouth. Improper usage of either the mouth or the tongue can lead to troubles which may broaden the spiritual distance between ourselves and Hashem.[7]

The importance of proper diet and good health care is literally doubled for the expectant mother. Nutritional intake during pregnancy directly affects the future health of the newborn. This is not a new scientific theory. It is advice which is given several times in the Talmud, an illustration of which is the discussion of Yishmael ben Kimchis. The Talmud tells us that he was able to hold 4 *kav* in his hand, a great volume. When asked to explain his great strength, he said that his mother, Kimchis, had eaten sprouts and a certain type of grain during pregnancy and this influenced his development.[8]

The story of Shimshon in the *Tanach* provides another example of how the future of the child is affected by what the mother eats. Shimshon was to be a *nazir* from the time of his conception: "For a *nazir* of God he will be from the womb." The angel therefore commanded his mother to abstain from wine, grapes, and all foods that are forbidden to a *nazir*. She was not told to observe the other restrictions of *nezirus*, such as cutting her hair and not becoming a *temeh mes* — only to refrain from those prohibitions which would have a direct influence on the fetus: i.e., the nourishment she provided through her diet.[9]

Our Sages did not rely on our ability to understand the important lesson to be learned from such stories. They clearly warn the pregnant mother against eating the wrong foods: "One who drinks intoxicating liquor during pregnancy will have ungainly children." They also promise sweet rewards to those who eat the right foods: "One who eats parsley will have beautiful children."[10]

Thus it is clear that the proper approach to diet during, and even before, pregnancy will yield very positive results in the health of our children.[11]

It is a common myth that proper diet means low fat and low calorie intake. There is more to good nutrition than that. Eating at the proper times, the correct amounts, and other basic dietary rules are just as important as what we eat.

Let us now explore some of the nutritional guidelines that *Chazal* have handed down to us.

While acknowledging the benefit of organizing and   **Digestion**
scheduling our activities, we should also recognize
the advantage of planning our daily diet and eating routine. Eating patterns should follow a strategy, and not
just be a reflex to hunger. A nutritious meal should provide maximum potential for strength and energy. It
should not produce negative side effects, such as an upset stomach or a sluggish feeling. A meal which does not
achieve these objectives fails to fulfill the requirements of
a nutritious meal.

The Rambam states that the primary goal of proper
nutrition is to insure efficient digestive function.[12] All of
our eating should be goal-oriented, supplying sufficient
vitamins and minerals and providing for optimum utilization of nutrients and the excretion of wastes.

The berachah, Asher Yatzar, recalls the wonders of
the digestive and excretory processes, ending with the
words: "Rofeh kol basar u'mafli la'asos — Who heals all
flesh and acts wondrously." We thus acknowledge that
Hashem has endowed man with the ability to choose
food that is good for the body, has created each part of
the body with the capacity to differentiate and assimilate
the nourishment specifically suitable for it, and finally,
empowered the body to reject and eliminate waste. For if
the waste should remain in the body, it would, God forbid, cause disease.[13]

In order to maintain a healthy and vigorous body, the
digestive system must function properly. It is important,
therefore, to plan a diet which enables good digestion.
This means eating at the right time, choosing foods
which are easily digested, avoiding overeating, keeping
bowel movements soft, and exercising regularly.[14] Ignor-
ing these principles can lead to constipation, heartburn,
gas, and even cancer of the colon or many other very serious diseases.[15]

A more detailed discussion of these principles follows.

Rav Acha bar Ya'akov said, "At first the Jews [in   **When to Eat**
the desert] were like chickens pecking at trash [eat-

ing at all times of the day], until Moshe came and designated the appropriate times to eat."[16]

A person should eat two meals a day,[17] except for Shabbos, when three meals are specified. The *halachah* of providing for the needy supports this recommendation, instructing us to give two meals a day as the basic requirement of daily sustenance.[18]

The best time for the first meal is from mid- to late morning.[19] A substantial meal should not be eaten immediately upon arising because the digestive system is not yet sufficiently invigorated to efficiently process the food. Eating a heavy meal before the digestive system has had a chance to "wake up" imposes a great strain on total body function. It is preferable to stimulate the system by doing some work or exercising before the first meal.[20]

We should not entirely skip eating first thing in the morning, as we need something to tide us over until our first meal. When we wake up, our blood glucose level is at rock bottom. Glucose, which is the end product of carbohydrate breakdown, fuels all body function, so a low morning blood sugar causes a strong feeling of hunger.

What to Eat   What should we eat early in the morning? The Rambam, along with many modern nutritionists, recommends eating fruit.[21] Breaking one's fast with fruit will satisfy the early morning appetite without weighing one down for the rest of the day. Fruit is naturally high in energy-producing fructose, which breaks down rapidly to glucose, raising our blood sugar level almost instantaneously. In addition to satisfying our body's glucose needs, fruit also provides the body with vitamins and minerals.

Joy Gross, author of *The Vegetarian Child*, refers to fruit as a "natural carbohydrate" because fruit's simple molecular chains of sugar are rapidly broken down and utilized in the body. Thus, eating fruit does not impose a heavy strain on the digestive system, as it is digested quickly and easily.[22]

Because of fruit's high water content, it passes rapidly through the stomach to be broken down in the intestines. In contrast, other foods take from six to eight hours to be partially digested in the stomach before they pass on to the intestines to be further assimilated.

The high water content of fruit not only enhances its own digestion, but also reinforces the ability of the intestines to digest other food. The combination of the fiber and the water in fruit lubricates the intestines, promoting peristalsis, the muscular contractions which aid the movement of food through the intestinal tract. Fruit, therefore, is a good assistant to the process of excretion, which the body usually handles in the early morning. Moreover, to load up with a big meal before the body has had a chance to "unload" is simply too much of a strain on the digestive system.

Fruit, therefore, is not only beneficial in appeasing morning hunger without burdening the system; it even furthers the digestive and excretory functions.

During pregnancy the digestive process is easily disrupted. The pressure of the growing uterus on the digestive organs, the hormonal influence reducing peristalsis in the intestines, iron supplements, and a lack of exercise all contribute to the disruption of normal digestion. As a result, constipation and hemorrhoids are common in pregnant women. Consequently, starting the day with fruit can only be of benefit.

Since fluctuations in blood sugar levels during pregnancy are so drastic, fruit may not be enough to satisfy your hunger in the early morning. Adding yogurt, granola or other *light* foods will provide a comfortable, full feeling until the first meal.

Low blood glucose is one of the contributing factors of morning sickness. Eating naturally sweet fruit, therefore, will help combat it. Avoiding extreme fluctuations in blood glucose levels is the key to preventing nausea in pregnancy. One can maintain consistent glucose levels by snacking on fruit or other nutritious foods.

FROM LIGHT TO HEAVY

The Rambam asserts that light foods should be eaten before heavy foods[23]: e.g., first eggs, then chicken, then meat. The purpose of this is to gradually expand the digestive tract. This theory does not only apply to one meal, but to the entire day's eating pattern. Light foods should be eaten at the beginning of the day, leading up to heavy foods at the end of the day.

Eating food in a specific order fulfills the simple but vital function of generating maximal energy for the body. Digestion is a lengthy process entailing an increased blood supply to the digestive organs and the utilization of a great deal of energy. That is why we were always told not to engage in strenuous activity on a full stomach.

"In the evening you shall eat meat and in the morning you shall be satisfied with bread."[24] The Talmud expounds on this verse, "Here the Torah teaches us *derech eretz*, that meat should only be eaten at night."[25] Rashi elaborates on the words of *Chazal*, adding another guideline: "Here the Torah teaches us *derech eretz*, that a person should not fill up on meat."[26]

Three very important rules of nutrition can be deduced from this verse and its interpretations:

1. One's main food source should be bread, as it is written, "Be satisfied with bread."

2. One should not eat large portions of meat, for although we are told to eat meat, we should not be satisfied with the meat (Rashi's emphasis).

3. Meat should be eaten only in the evening, as it is written, "In the evening you shall eat meat" (Talmud's emphasis).

Let us discuss these three principles which should guide our daily eating pattern:

BREAD: Bread should be the main substance of our diet. For this reason *birkas ha-mazon* was instituted for bread and not for other foods. Recently, nutritionists have begun to realize that bread and grains should comprise the major part of our diet.

SMALL PORTIONS OF MEAT: Meat is a fine source of protein (as will be discussed later). But how much of a portion do we need? A recent article in *Newsweek* on proper nutrition states: "The half pound sirloin in the center of the plate carries nearly one and a half times the amount of protein one needs in a whole day, and it is packed with saturated fat [that can lead to cancer]. The excess protein can be fattening as well."[27] *Chazal* always considered meat or fish a *davar le'lapes es ha-pas*[28] — a condiment to the bread (or grain). Meat was never meant to be a main course.

MEAT IN THE EVENING: Rashi interprets the injunction not to fill up on meat as a warning to decrease the size of our meat portions. He does not mean that we should only partake of a little meat and then leave the table hungry. Everyone wants to feel full in the evening. Surely Rashi's intention is that we should be satisfied from bread in the evening, as we are during the day, but also add a little meat to accompany the staple bread and grains.[29]

The experience of eating a heavy meal and feeling its sleep-inducing effects helps us to understand why we are advised to eat this type of meal in the evening. (In many societies where the main meal is eaten midday, shops, offices and businesses routinely close during afternoon hours to allow people to sleep off their meal.) The evening provides a natural opportunity to unwind, and therefore is most conducive for a heavier meal. Even if one is a bit tired when the meal is over, the reduced energy level will still suffice to fulfill the evening's lighter demands. One should also be careful to time the second meal early enough in the evening to avoid going to bed on a full stomach, as it is unhealthy to sleep soon after eating. [30]

In summary, the first meal of the day should be filling and satisfying, yet not divert one's entire energy to digestion. A menu based on carbohydrates (bread/grains) and vegetables would, therefore, be most appropriate.[31] It is well known that vegetables are an excellent source of vitamins and minerals, so much so that vegetables are considered a good component of any meal. *Chazal* praised the nutritional value of vegetables and even declared that a *talmid chacham* should not live in a city that does not have vegetables.[32] In the Torah, vegetables are called "*oros* — lights," for they light up our eyes.[33]

The second meal should be eaten in the late afternoon/early evening,[34] or about 6-8 hours after the first meal, corresponding to the amount of time required for digestion.[35] For this meal a menu of bread/grain and a protein as a side dish is suggested.[36]

Additional Meals in Pregnancy   Though we advocate eating two meals a day, certain circumstances, such as illness, cause digestive disturbances which prevent adherence to this diet. The Rambam agrees that when conditions are not favorable, it is permissible for a person to stray from his regular dietary plan.[37] And the *Mishnah Berurah* even recommends that a weak person eat more than two meals a day.[38]

Pregnant women are often advised to eat small, frequent meals to help cope with occasional symptoms of nausea or heartburn.[39] If one is pregnant and suffering from digestive disorders, she should not feel bound by this diet. When the pregnant woman has no stomach complaints, however, it is recommended that she eat as has been suggested.

In order to know more about what to eat, we must understand the composition of food and how it affects the body. We will now explain how protein, iron, calcium, vitamins, fat, salt, fluids, and carbohydrates fit into our daily diet and are essential for the well-being of both mother and baby.

Protein   The primary function of protein in the body is to promote cellular structure and growth, not to provide energy. Protein is composed of amino acids, which act as building blocks and are responsible for chemical reactions and adding structure to individual cells. In order to utilize the protein, the body breaks it down into amino acids.

There are 22 different types of amino acids, eight of which cannot be manufactured in the body and must be obtained from the food we eat. These eight are referred to as "essential amino acids." A food is called a "complete protein" when it contains all eight essential amino acids.[40]

Providing the body with sufficient protein is especially important during pregnancy, when the mother is supplying the protein needed for cellular growth and tissue repair for both herself and her growing baby. While the development of all body systems and the function of the placenta are dependent on protein, the fetus requires protein particularly for the proper formation of the brain and nervous system.

Protein requirements, however, are quite paradoxical. On the one hand, one must eat a minimum of protein to support body functions. On the other hand, excessive protein intake can lead to high cholesterol and increase the risk of heart disease.[41] The average woman of childbearing age needs 44 gr. of protein per day and an additional 30 gr. during pregnancy.[42]

One should carefully choose from among a variety of protein sources. Protein intake from meat sources can raise cholesterol in the bloodstream, as well as cause vascular diseases. For these reasons, although meat products have been widely touted as complete proteins, they should be eaten in moderation. A woman need not, however, worry about cholesterol intake during pregnancy unless her doctor instructs her to do so.

Protein can easily be acquired from non-meat sources such as peanut butter, split peas, brown rice and whole wheat. Certain non-meat protein foods can be combined to form a complete protein, e.g., beans eaten with rice. Another suggestion for the use of complimentary proteins is to substitute part of the wheat flour with soy flour when baking.

A Guide to Daily Food Choices

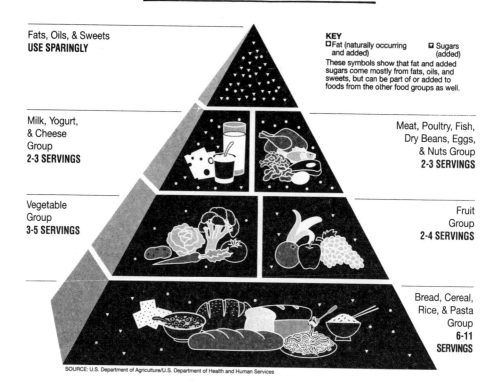

Fats, Oils, & Sweets
USE SPARINGLY

KEY
☐Fat (naturally occurring and added)   ☑ Sugars (added)
These symbols show that fat and added sugars come mostly from fats, oils, and sweets, but can be part of or added to foods from the other food groups as well.

Milk, Yogurt, & Cheese Group
2-3 SERVINGS

Meat, Poultry, Fish, Dry Beans, Eggs, & Nuts Group
2-3 SERVINGS

Vegetable Group
3-5 SERVINGS

Fruit Group
2-4 SERVINGS

Bread, Cereal, Rice, & Pasta Group
6-11 SERVINGS

SOURCE: U.S. Department of Agriculture/U.S. Department of Health and Human Services

WHAT COUNTS AS A SERVING?

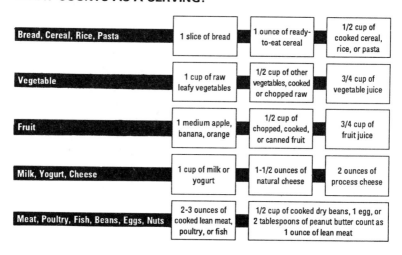

Bread, Cereal, Rice, Pasta	1 slice of bread	1 ounce of ready-to-eat cereal	1/2 cup of cooked cereal, rice, or pasta
Vegetable	1 cup of raw leafy vegetables	1/2 cup of other vegetables, cooked or chopped raw	3/4 cup of vegetable juice
Fruit	1 medium apple, banana, orange	1/2 cup of chopped, cooked, or canned fruit	3/4 cup of fruit juice
Milk, Yogurt, Cheese	1 cup of milk or yogurt	1-1/2 ounces of natural cheese	2 ounces of process cheese
Meat, Poultry, Fish, Beans, Eggs, Nuts	2-3 ounces of cooked lean meat, poultry, or fish	1/2 cup of cooked dry beans, 1 egg, or 2 tablespoons of peanut butter count as 1 ounce of lean meat	

The soybean is an inexpensive and healthy source of protein. Soybean products are available as packaged products, inexpensive soy chips (SVP) or tofu. Tofu, like other soy products, contains an abundance of lysine, an essential amino acid that is deficient in many grain products.[43]

Vegetarianism and Pregnancy

It is possible for vegetarians to consume adequate supplies of protein, but this requires taking extra time in planning and preparing meals. One must take care not to lose more nutritionally than one benefits from being vegetarian. Many pregnant vegetarians turn to meat and fish because they feel weak and malnourished on an improperly balanced vegetarian diet.

The National Academy of Sciences cautions that, "The most important safeguard for the average [vegetarian] consumer is variety in the diet."[44] It is critical for the vegetarian to cook creatively, choosing from a variety of foods that will prevent deficiency, not only in the area of protein, but in all areas of nutrition.

Iron

Iron manifests itself in the body as hemoglobin in the blood. Hemoglobin enables oxygen to be supplied throughout the body. Therefore, a low hemoglobin level can cause fatigue and pallor. No matter how high a woman's hemoglobin level is at the beginning of pregnancy, it will drop by the third trimester, adding to the feeling of fatigue. Blood loss at delivery further depletes a woman's iron stores.

Maintaining iron at the appropriate level is important for mother as well as baby. For the first three months of life, the baby's iron needs are sustained by the iron assimilated during intrauterine life and stored in the baby's liver. Your baby is counting on you! The iron requirement for an adult woman is 18 mg. per day, with an additional 30-60 mg. needed during pregnancy.[45]

Iron is found in abundance in liver, red meat, eggs, beans, leafy green vegetables, peas, cornmeal, watermelon, dried fruit, and whole wheat. Six slices of whole wheat bread, for example, supply half a day's iron requirement.

Many women take iron supplements during pregnancy. An iron supplement usually consists of folic acid, which prevents megaloblastic anemia (folic acid deficiency). Folic acid works together with Vitamin B_{12} to maintain the normal development and metabolism of blood cells in the bone marrow. Low levels of folic acid may be associated with premature separation of the placenta or spontaneous abortion.[46]

Supplements are needed only if hemoglobin levels fall to 12.6 or below. Iron supplements can cause black stools and constipation in some women. Certain brands of iron supplements cause more stomach upset than others. Therefore, if you have any digestive disturbances, your doctor can prescribe a different brand of supplement which may better agree with your system. For optimum iron absorption, take any iron supplement with orange juice (Vitamin C), and not with dairy products.

Calcium   In addition to protein and iron, calcium is especially important in a woman's diet. Nutritionists recommend a daily intake of 800 mg. of calcium. During pregnancy, however, an additional 400 mg.[47] is essential for the formation of the baby's skeleton and teeth as well as for proper maintenance of the mother's body. The fetus will take the calcium it needs from the mother's body, often rendering her calcium-depleted and -deficient.

Calcium deficiency can cause dental problems and skeletal changes resulting in osteoporosis (brittle bones). All women are therefore cautioned to maintain an optimum dietary intake of calcium, not only during pregnancy, but throughout their lives.

In addition to dairy products, foods offering an abundance of calcium are: leafy green vegetables, nuts, citrus fruits, and sesame seeds.

Vitamins   Vitamins are used in the body to promote good health and sustain metabolic processes. Increased vitamin and mineral requirements during pregnancy are generally satisfied by eating a well-balanced diet chosen from a variety of foods. Vitamin supplements are helpful in the event of dietary deficiencies, but it is much better to eat well than to rely on supplementation.

A new Institute of Medicine report says that there is no convincing evidence to show the benefits of vitamin supplements in women who ate a balanced diet. Another study revealed that although there were a significantly lower number of birth defects when mothers took daily multivitamin supplements during the first six weeks of pregnancy, no benefits were noted when vitamins were taken after the sixth week of pregnancy.[48]

Excessive vitamin supplements are dangerous, whether or not one is pregnant. Megadoses of vitamins can threaten the health of the fetus, especially in the case of fat-soluble vitamins (A, D, E, and K), which are not easily excreted. Too much Vitamin A can cause birth defects such as bone deformities, and excessive Vitamin D can lead to kidney problems. Even though water soluble vitamins (B and C) are more easily eliminated through the urine, megadoses are still unsafe for the expectant mother and her baby.[49]

If you suspect a vitamin deficiency or would like to continue your present vitamin supplement, consult your doctor.

Fat

Fat, which is composed of fatty acids, plays an important role in the synthesis of many hormones — most importantly, estrogen. This is illustrated by the cessation of the menses (period) as a result of starvation or extreme dieting. It should therefore never be totally eliminated from the diet.

An overabundance of animal fat has proven to be detrimental to our health. Numerous studies show that populations consuming a high-fat diet (especially rich in meat and dairy products) have a higher rate of certain cancers. The National Cancer Institute, the American Cancer Society, and the National Academy of Sciences have all recognized the possible role of dietary fat in cancer and recommend reducing fat intake to help prevent cancer.[50]

Yet fat from vegetable sources — e.g., olive oil, canola oil, various nut oils — is beneficial in our diet. It is recommended that fat should comprise no more than 30% of our dietary intake.[51]

Salt   Salt is comprised of sodium chloride, which acts as a water regulator in our body. Too much sodium in the body will lead to fluid retention (edema) and a lack of sodium, caused by sweating or excessive urination, can result in dehydration and weakness. Since so much of our food already contains salt, it is usually unnecessary to add salt at the table. However, it is not necessary to restrict salt during pregnancy, unless so advised by one's physician.[52]

Fluids   It is just as important to monitor our fluid intake as it is to eat the proper foods. A proportionately high fluid intake is vital to general health maintenance. As 70% of the body is composed of water, there are those who advocate that 70% of our diet should be in liquid form or in the form of food with high water content, such as fruits and vegetables.[53]

The *Kitzur Shulchan Aruch* tells us that, "Clean, pure water aids the body to preserve moisture and hastens the elimination of wastes."[54]

Water gives form to the human body, supports metabolic processes, and helps to maintain body temperature. Liquids are also necessary to prevent constipation and promote regular bowel movements. Approximately 75% of fecal material is water.[55]

Knowing when to drink is also important to maintaining one's health. The Rambam warns against drinking together with a meal and advises that we drink only after the food starts to be digested. It seems to be a basic rule in nutrition that drinking while eating interrupts digestion and the absorption of food. However, the Rambam does permit drinking a small quantity of water or wine during a meal. He generally recommends that a person drink only when thirsty.[56]

Just as the amount of food we require fluctuates according to the seasons of the year, so, too, do our fluid requirements. The Rambam suggests that during the summer we decrease our food intake by one third.[57] On the other hand, fluid intake should be increased during the summer. In winter we need about eight glasses of water or fruit juice per day, while during the summer months, twelve glasses per day are recommended to insure adequate fluid intake. It is good to make a habit of drinking a glass of liquid every waking hour in the summer.

A pregnant mother is drinking for two, so she must make an even greater effort to drink adequately. Milk and natural juices may be substituted for water, but one should avoid soda or sweetened drinks, which merely add gas and chemicals to the body.

Pregnant women and nursing mothers should think of themselves as constantly being thirsty. Excessive drinking will never go to waste as all fluid intake is used to support body processes. Extra fluids are needed for the kidneys to function, and the pregnant woman must endure the added strain of excreting both her own and her baby's wastes.

Dehydration, which can lead to premature contractions, is all too common in pregnant women, for although they may think they are drinking enough, in reality they should be drinking even more.

Carbohydrates

Last but not least is the friend or foe of our diet, carbohydrates. Carbohydrates comprise the bulk of our diet — about 50-60% of our daily intake. The body breaks carbohydrates down to glucose, supplying energy and thus reserving protein for its job of growth and repair.

When we think of carbohydrates, we instantly think of "junk food." Eating carbohydrates, however, does not necessarily mean consuming fattening, empty calories. It depends on the type of carbohydrates one eats.

Carbohydrates are molecules of sugars and starches linked together. When the sugar-starch chain is disrupted (for example, in the excessive processing of junk foods), fiber is eliminated and thus the foods are less filling. When full satisfaction is denied, one is left with the desire to eat even more. Calories are consumed without nutritional benefit, ultimately resulting in a total neglect of proper eating habits and a disregard for higher quality foods. Furthermore, these overprocessed carbohydrates are difficult to digest, and their breakdown produces considerable waste and leaves many extra calories behind in the body. It is for these reasons that carbohydrates have acquired the reputation of being very fattening.

Natural carbohydrates — such as potatoes, whole wheat bread, unprocessed fruits, vegetables and grains — are easily broken down into glucose to fuel the body. In addition to energy, they supply us with a host of nutrients. The body utilizes many components of these natural carbohydrates. Therefore less waste and calories remain in the body when we assimilate these than when we consume the overprocessed carbohydrates. What's more, despite common misconceptions, one would have to eat a huge amount of plain cooked potatoes to really gain weight. Frying, buttering, and smothering the potato with cheese and ketchup is what makes it fattening.

With regard to bread, eating a smaller quantity of whole wheat bread provides more nutritional benefits and a fuller feeling than filling up on plain white bread. Whole wheat also contains bran, which has been removed from all white bleached flour. Although bran is getting a great deal of publicity due to modern nutritional research, its importance is not a new health food concept. The *Kitzur Shulchan Aruch* says, "Because fine flour takes too long to digest, it should contain some bran."[58] Bran contains fiber which enhances the bowel function and prevents constipation.

Generally speaking, whole wheat flour is nutritionally richer than processed white flour. The *Kitzur Shulchan Aruch* describes white flour as unwholesome: "One should not eat too much of fine flour which has been so thoroughly sifted that even a morsel of bran has disappeared."[59] It is difficult to discern the original grain of wheat in the typical snack treat which has been stabilized, emulsified, preserved, sweetened, salted, colored Sunset Yellow, and coated with chemicals such as E-122.

In every nutrient category, whole wheat bread, pasta, brown rice, and whole grains are more nutritionally beneficial than their processed counterparts. Moreover, the fact that they are also more filling makes their use economical.

In conclusion, it is easy to see that Hashem provided us with food products which are most beneficial in their natural, unprocessed state.

Food can be enhanced through creative preparation, but we must take care not to totally strip it of its nutritional and life-sustaining benefits. This is an abuse of the food resources Hashem has given us. We should choose foods which provide the greatest possible nutritional benefit.

The Rambam admonishes us to eat healthy foods, not merely the foods we like. An even harsher approach to eating the wrong foods is found in the Ra'avad's *Ba'alei Ha-Nefesh*:

> There are two reasons to avoid eating harmful foods. First, to prevent the food from causing physical harm. Second, to humble the *yetzer ha-ra* and break his cravings... because certainly a person must be careful not to eat foods which he knows are bad for him. Someone who eats harmful and unnecessary foods is criminally abusing his body and soul. He is swayed by his cravings and disregards the deterioration caused to his body. This is the method the *yetzer ha-ra* uses to entice him to stray from the path of life to that of death.[60]

Eating low-quality junk food may be a quick remedy for hunger, but in the long run will only serve to weaken our bodies and cause illness.

Overeating How much we eat is just as important to maintaining health as when and what we eat. The Rambam emphasizes that eating too much is detrimental to our health, even if it is nutritionally wholesome food: "Overeating is the drug of death. Most sickness is a direct result of overeating. Even an excess of healthful foods can make one sick."[61]

So we see that overeating can be compared to overdosing on drugs. The results of overeating can make us sick for days, not to mention the long term consequences of weight gain and disease associated with poor eating habits.

The unpleasant feeling caused by overeating is a sign that the digestive system is overburdened with food it cannot handle. Gas passes through the digestive tract and is trapped in the intestines, which are so full that they cannot even absorb nutrients or water. Diarrhea, the body's attempt to flush out the system, is often a side effect of overeating. Thus, even if good foods are consumed in excess, their potential nutrients will be lost in the body's effort to eliminate the surplus.

Overeating can create a cycle of detrimental effects. Habitual overeating results in the overproduction of stomach acid (heartburn), which creates a dependency on antacid medication. Antacids can cause constipation, which may necessitate even more medication. Thus, if not interrupted, this pattern can easily lead to ulcers and other digestive diseases.

The Rambam, who recommends moderation, tells us not to eat until we are so full that we feel stuffed, but only until we are three-quarters full.[62] According to the *Kitzur Shulchan Aruch*, a person should eat only when he has a natural hunger for food and not an indulgent desire.[63] When pregnant, indulging one's cravings for certain foods should not be used as an excuse to overeat.

One should clearly differentiate between the psychological desire for food and the physical requirements of nourishment.

A pregnant woman, who might not be feeling quite up to par, may justify her indulgence in "something special." Unfortunately, cravings usually result in overeating fattening, low quality foods, not fruits and vegetables. The fetus will not gain from this kind of eating, but her hips will!

Extra weight gain in pregnancy puts an even greater strain on the heart and muscular-skeletal structures. It also causes a predisposition to high blood pressure and diabetes. Moreover, weight gain other than that needed to support the pregnancy is much harder to lose after the birth, especially in medium and large-boned women.

It takes a great deal of willpower and self-discipline to avoid overeating, but the benefits to be derived are clear. Pregnancy is not the time to neglect good dietary habits. It is rather a time to especially adhere to the principles of good nutrition. The continued good health of the mother, her baby, and the entire family is an added incentive to embrace proper eating habits.

The undertaking of a healthier and more natural lifestyle is often bound together with a person's quest for broader spiritual fulfillment. The decision to lead a healthier life is the first step in *teshuvah*. As Rabbi Avraham Yitzchak Kook wrote:

> Natural repentance is comprised of physical and spiritual aspects. Physical repentance encompasses all transgressions against the laws of nature, as well as against the moral conscience and Torah which are bound up with the laws of nature. The result of all evil conduct is sickness and pain, and the individual as well as society suffer intensely on account of it. Once a person clearly realizes that he is himself responsible for the deterioration of his life strength, he will undertake to rectify the situation and will turn back to the laws of life and abide by the laws of nature, ethics, and Torah, so that he may return and live. And then life will be restored to him in all its vigor.[64]

NOTES

1. Rambam, *Hilchos De'os* 4:1.
2. For if a person could have lived until the age of 70, but due to his high cholesterol and blood pressure, his life was cut short twenty years, then twenty years of mitzvos were forfeited. "Better one hour of repentance and good deeds in this world than the entire life of the World-to-Come" (*Pirkei Avos* 4:22).
3. *Shabbos* 129a. Rav and Shemuel both said that if one is indifferent to eating a meal after bloodletting, then Hashem will likewise be indifferent regarding his nutritional needs (*mezonos*). "He who did not take pity on his own life, why should I take pity on him?"
4. *Vayikra Rabbah*, 34:3.
5. Rambam, *Hilchos De'os* 4:15; *see also* Carper, *Brand Name Nutrition Counter* (New York: Bantam Books, 1985), p. 19.
6. *Mishlei* 21:23.
7. Rambam, *Hilchos De'os* 4:15 — maybe that is why the Rambam included his *halachos* on health care in the section of *Mishneh Torah* in which he taught the laws of *shemiras ha-lashon.*
8. *Yoma* 47a.
9. *Shoftim* 13:4; *see Musar Ha-Nevi'im* (Feldheim).
10. *Kesubbos* 60; other examples can be found there as well.
11. *Yoma* 47a, the story of Reb Yishmael ben Kimchis (*ikka d'amrei*).
12. Rambam, *Hilchos De'os* 4:13.
13. *Kitzur Shulchan Aruch* 32:2.
14. Rambam, *Hilchos De'os* 4:2, 6, 13, 14.
15. B. Long, W. Phipps, and N. Woods, *Medical-Surgical Nursing* (St. Louis: C.V. Mosby Co., 1979), p. 1244.
16. *Yoma* 75b.
17. *Kitzur Shulchan Aruch* 32:10; *Shemos* 16:8.
18. *Yoreh De'ah* 253:1; *see* Taz.
19. Maharsha, *Yoma* 75b; *see* Hebrew appendix.
20. Rambam, *Hilchos De'os* 4:2.
21. Rambam, ibid. 4:6; however, the Rambam makes a distinction between watery fruits that are easy to digest, and other fruits such as apples which he does not recommend.
22. J. Gross, *The Vegetarian Child* (Secaucus, N.J.: Lyle Stuart Inc., 1983), pp. 42-48.
23. Rambam, *Hilchos De'os* 4:7.
24. *Shemos* 16:8.
25. *Yoma* 75b.
26. Rashi, *Shemos* 16:8; *see Mishnah Berurah* 157:4 and *Kaf Ha-Chayim* 157:37, 38.

27. C. Koel, L. Shapiro, et al., "Food Frenzy," *Newsweek*, May 27, 1991, pp. 42-48.
28. For example, see *Shulchan Aruch, Orach Chayim* 291:5.
29. *Siftei Chachamim* on Rashi, 16:8 (*Otzar Mefarshei Rashi*).
30. Rambam, *Hilchos De'os* 4:5.
31. See *Mishnah Berurah* 157:4.
32. *Eruvin*, 55b.
33. Rashi and Radak, *Melachim II*, 4:39.
34. See *Kaf Ha-Chayim* 157:37, 38.
35. B. Landau, *Essential Human Anatomy and Physiology* (Glenview, Ill: Scott, Foresman Co., 1980), p. 573.
36. The *Mishnah Berurah* and *Kaf Ha-Chayim* also recommend that we adhere to the guidance of *Chazal* in regard to these principles of nutrition (157).
37. Rambam, *Hilchos De'os* 4:21.
38. *Mishnah Berurah*, 157:4.
39. Willis and Foster, *Human Nutrition* (New York: McGraw Hill, 1988).
40. B. Landau, *Essential Human Anatomy and Physiology*, p. 600.
41. Health Almanac, *U.S. News and World Report*, 1991.
42. Food and Nutrition Board, Recommended Daily Dietary Allowances, National Academy of Sciences.
43. W. Shurteff and A. Aoyagi, *Book of Tofu*, (New York: Ballantine Books, 1975), p. 23.
44. J. Gross, *The Vegetarian Child* (Secaucus, N.J.: Lyle Stuart Inc., 1983), p. 94.
45. Food and Nutrition Board, Recommended Daily Dietary Allowances, National Academy of Sciences.
46. D.C. Knab, "Abruptio Placentae: An Assessment of the Time and Method of Delivery," *Obstetrics and Gynecology*, (1978) 52:625.
47. Food and Nutrition Board, Recommended Daily Dietary Allowances, National Academy of Sciences.
48. Health Almanac, *U.S. News and World Report*, June 1990.
49. Ibid.
50. J. Carper, *Brand Name Nutrition Counter* (New York: Bantam, 1985), p. 19.
51. U.S.D.A. and U.S. Department of Health and Human Services, 1990 Dietary Guidelines.
52. Pilliteri, *Maternal-Newborn Nursing* (Boston: Little Brown & Co., 1981), p. 246.
53. H. Diamond & M. Diamond, *Fit for Life*, (New York: Warner Books, 1985), p. 581.
54. *Kitzur Shulchan Aruch* 32:17.

55. B. Landau, *Essential Human Anatomy and Physiology*, p. 581.

56. *Kitzur Shulchan Aruch* 32:17; Rambam, *Hilchos De'os* 4:2; *Newsweek*, May 27, 1991 presents a theory that drinking wine with meals helps prevent certain diseases. With this theory we can try to answer the Maharsha's question on Rashi in *Bava Metzia* 107b; Rashi, "*Pat Ba-Melach.*"

57. Rambam, *Hilchos De'os*, 4:12.

58. *Kitzur Shulchan Aruch* 32:17.

59. Ibid. 32:16.

60. Ra'avad, *Ba'alei Ha-Nefesh* (Mossad Ha-Rav Kook), ch. *Sha'ar Ha-Kedushah*, pp. 125-126; *see* Hebrew appendix.

61. Rambam, *Hilchos De'os*, 4:16.

62. Rambam, ibid. 4:2; *see Fit for Life*, p. 187.

63. *Kitzur Shulchan Aruch* 4:10.

64. *Oros Ha-Teshuvah*, ch. 1.

9 | Fitness and Exercise

...They shall mount up with wings as
eagles; they shall run and not be weary;
they shall walk and not faint.
YESHAYAHU 40:31

As we discussed previously, one of the Rambam's fundamental principles for maintaining good health is exercise. The Rambam warns us that inactivity can make a person ill or weak, especially when combined with improper eating and elimination.[1]

Modern authorities also concur that exercise is a necessary prerequisite to healthy living, whether a woman is pregnant or not.[2] Exercise causes endorphins to be released in the body. Endorphins are chemicals generated by the brain, which produce effects similar to opiates (e.g., pain relief). This explains the "natural high" one feels after exercising, as well as the easing of minor aches and pains.

Before the baby is born, exercise will prepare you for labor and delivery; while after birth, it is critical to repair and restrengthen the body. In addition to the psychological benefits of exercise, we thus find that exercise during pregnancy is a physiological imperative.

Recent research demonstrates that regular moderate exercise helps to prevent bone loss from osteoporosis, particularly in women over 30.[3] It has been shown that calcium is more readily absorbed and utilized by the bones if accompanied by exercise. This is especially significant for pregnant and postpartum women, who have a greater need for calcium.

Exercising *now*, whatever your stage of childbearing, will promote good health in the present and prevent impairment of body function in the future.

Exercise Guidelines   Before beginning any exercise program, your doctor should be consulted. No matter what your exercise routine is, you should become aware of the guidelines to prevent injury. Not all pregnant women are alike, and each trimester of pregnancy imposes different restrictions. As the uterus increases in size, many activities become more difficult. Listen to your body. When it becomes stiff and inflexible, it is telling you that you are overworking it.

A woman should be able to continue with any exercise activities that she enjoyed before becoming pregnant, but pregnancy is not the time to take up new sports. Your sense of balance is off due to softened ligaments that can make pregnant women more prone to falls and injury. Therefore, it is recommended to avoid strenuous and competitive sports during pregnancy. Vigorous bouncing can overstretch the ligaments in the feet, knees, hips and vertebrae, causing permanent joint instability.

❧ Do not exercise immediately after eating. The Rambam advises exercising before a meal.[4]

❧ Drink before, during and after exercise to prevent dehydration.

❧ Avoid exercising in the heat of the day, and never use saunas, steam rooms, and hot tubs. When temperature increases dramatically, the body will try to cool off by diverting blood away from the uterus to the skin.

❧ Wear cool, comfortable clothes when exercising.

❧ Wear well-cushioned shoes.

❦ If you begin to sweat profusely, stop exercising.

❦ Do not remain on your back for more than 4 minutes at a time.

AEROBICS

Aerobics can be a part of any exercise routine. Aerobic exercise simply means exercising with oxygen (meaning, proper breathing), which can take many forms: brisk walking, swimming, or dancing.

The increased heart rate resulting from exercise will benefit overall circulation and strengthen all the muscles in your body, including the heart. The American College of Obstetrics and Gynecology advises all pregnant women to take care to keep their heart rate below 140 beats per minute. If a woman chooses aerobic activity to maintain physical fitness during pregnancy, it is recommended that she limit herself to low intensity (heart rate elevated to 120-130 beats per minute) and low-impact (at least one foot on the floor at all times) aerobics. Aerobic exercise for a minimum of 20 minutes, three times a week is thought to be the most effective routine for attaining and maintaining physical fitness.

Exercise Programs

WALKING

Brisk walking is a free and easy way to exercise. It will get the heart pumping and the blood flowing. Be careful to restrict your walks to the cooler early morning or evening hours.

SWIMMING

Swimming is an all-around great way to exercise. Balance is not a problem, and all the body's muscles are exercised without strain. A woman may swim throughout her pregnancy as long as the amniotic membranes are intact, but she should avoid jumping or diving into the water, which can be traumatic to the uterus.

EXERCISE CLASSES

Exercise classes given by a certified instructor trained in prenatal and postnatal physiology offer the best opportunity to receive specialized exercise instruction. Exercising in an organized setting will motivate you to consistently attend and give you a chance to meet new people who share many of the same concerns about pregnancy and childbirth that you do.

Proper Body Mechanics   Two major goals of prenatal exercise include: maintenance of proper body mechanics and stretching and strengthening the muscles.

Correct posture and body alignment while standing, sitting and lying down are essential to prevent muscle strain and general discomfort. Most nonpregnant women should inculcate these principles and then learn to readjust them to fit the needs of pregnancy.

In addition to being a bad habit, faulty posture often indicates that you are feeling tired and unwell. Posture is the body's language for communicating to others how you are feeling. Holding your head high, standing tall and looking lively shows you feel good!

During pregnancy, posture must be adjusted to compensate for the force of gravity and the need to rebalance the body in response to the growing uterus and the softening of the ligaments. The "stance of pregnancy" — pelvis and hips jutting forward, body weight concentrated on the heels of the feet — hollows out the back, increasing backache and fatigue. Wearing high heels during pregnancy is not recommended, as they further undermine our posture and balance.

According to Elizabeth Noble in her book *Essential Exercises for the Childbearing Year*, good posture while standing is an ongoing process.[5] Tilt the pelvis in a relaxed position by tucking the buttocks down and under. Keep the shoulders straight and knees slightly bent. "Think tall" and hold your head high. Practice in front of a mirror, maintaining the proper posture for ten sec-

onds, and then relax. According to Noble, standing can
be a relaxing and endurance-building exercise routine.

Exercise 1: Posture

Stand with arms at your sides, palms facing forward, back to
the wall and feet a few inches away from it. Let your head,
shoulders and buttocks touch the wall. Press back your shoulders and trunk — but not the knees — and flatten out the
curves in your neck and lower back. Bring your arms upward
to your ears, then to shoulder level, and finally down again.
Repeat 5-10 times.

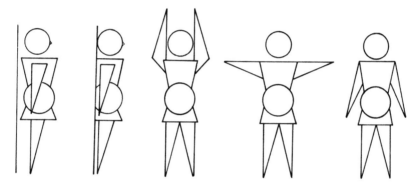

POSTURE AND MOVEMENT

Life does not stop once you are pregnant. You continue to bend, stretch, and change positions, not to
mention doing the taxing chores of housework and child-
care. You should always bear in mind that incorrect posture and uncoordinated movements can strain muscles
and cause temporary or even permanent damage. Adopt-
ing the fundamentals of proper movement will prevent
muscle strain and actually turn many of your daily activities into muscle-strengthening exercises.

▶ When lifting or working on floor level, do not bend
from the back. Squatting, with support if necessary, is a
functional position which stretches the muscles of the
pelvic floor and quadricep muscles (in the thighs).

▸ When lifting an object off the floor, always keep your knees bent so that they bear the load, instead of your back.

▸ Get down on your knees or on all fours when cleaning house or playing with the kids.

▸ Take the proper precautions when rising from a prone position in order to prevent strain on the abdominal muscles and on the uterine and ovarian ligaments. Bend both knees, roll to one side and push with your arms to achieve a sitting position. Only then should you stand up. This will also prevent the dizzy or faint feeling which sometimes accompanies sudden changes of position.

POSTURE IN SITTING — DOS AND DON'TS

▸ Elevate your feet whenever possible. Make sure that your calves are also supported. Rotate and stretch your feet to keep the blood circulating.

▸ Avoid sitting with knees crossed. This interferes with proper circulation and can cause varicose veins. Allow your legs to gently spread, and make sure that your knees are not higher than your hips.

▸ Sit back in the chair and avoid slumping, a position notorious in pregnancy. Use a cushion to help support the small of your back.

PRONE POSITION

So many of us enjoy resting and sleeping on our stomachs, and it is good to know that with proper positioning we can continue to do so during pregnancy. Several pillows will keep a big belly from interfering with comfort. Place one or two pillows under the hips (not under the abdomen) to raise the pelvis slightly and flatten the back. This relaxes the abdominal muscles and relieves back strain. Another pillow under the head is optional.

After delivery, lying on your stomach relieves discomfort from stitches and creates the proper pelvic tilt to facilitate the return of the pelvic organs to their original positions. It's comfortable and it feels good.

POSTURE WHILE LYING ON YOUR SIDE

Lying on your left side is a comfortable and healthy way to relax and sleep. In this position, your baby will receive optimal circulation and you will be able to breathe easily. By placing pillows beneath your head and abdomen and one lengthwise between your legs you will be most comfortable.

During pregnancy and after delivery, the muscles of the abdomen, back, and pelvic floor require special attention. These are the specific muscle areas which are stretched and strained most during pregnancy.

Strengthening the Muscles

ABDOMEN AND BACK

Though the muscles of the abdomen and back are on opposing sides of the body, they are closely related. When abdominal muscles are flabby and loose, the pain and discomfort resulting from their lax state will be felt in the lower back. The abdominal muscles maintain the proper position of the abdominal and pelvic organs (including the enlarging uterus). When abdominal muscles lose their tone, the burden of carrying the pregnancy and maintaining proper posture falls on the back muscles, leading to muscle strain and backache.

At the onset of labor, the abdominal muscles need to be relaxed, while in the second stage of labor these same muscles are required to contract in order to facilitate pushing. These multi-faceted functions of support, contraction and relaxation can be successfully achieved only through exercise.

The abdominal muscles form an elaborate network, which is stretched out during pregnancy and then needs exercise to regain its former tone. If muscle tone is not regained between pregnancies, the muscles will only stretch further, resulting in a protruding stomach and, in many cases, a chronic backache. A protruding stomach may become the most noticeable and "outstanding" feature of your body! To prevent this, begin the abdominal exercises — even during pregnancy.

According to Leora Ashkenazi, a certified fitness professional, shortening the abdominal muscles and lengthening the back muscles is considered a primary fitness goal. Only through simple, yet proper exercise can we tighten and tone the muscles in the abdomen and stretch overworked back muscles.

BEFORE YOU START

Prior to beginning an exercise routine — whether before, during, or after pregnancy — it is necessary to evaluate the condition of the abdominal muscles. We specifically examine the recti muscles which vertically extend along the midline of the abdomen in two halves, right and left. See illustration below.

The recti muscles may separate as a result of stress, similar to a zipper popping open. You will not feel this in the stomach, but you may feel a backache. If the recti muscles are already separated, you should avoid exercises which cause the gap to widen. The separation can be repaired in a matter of weeks by doing specific exercises on a regular basis. If you find no separation of the recti muscles, you may continue with the regular exercise routine to tighten and tone the abdominals.

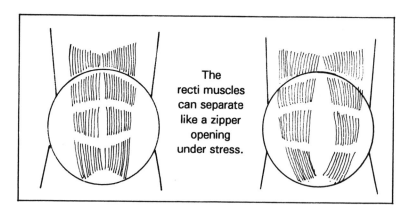

The recti muscles can separate like a zipper opening under stress.

SELF-CHECK FOR SEPARATION OF RECTI MUSCLES

Lying on your back, with knees bent, slowly raise your head and shoulders so that your neck is 8 inches off the floor.

Before the 4th month and postpartum: Place your fingers below the navel in the gap between the two sides of the recti muscles. A 1-2-finger-wide gap will tighten with regular exercise. A 3-4-finger gap or more requires special separation repair.

Advanced pregnancy: After raising your head, you will feel a bulge in the central abdominal area above the umbilicus. If the bulge is three fingers or more in width, the special separation repair exercise is needed.

Exercise 2: Curl-ups
Special Exercise for Separation Repair — Prenatal And Postpartum

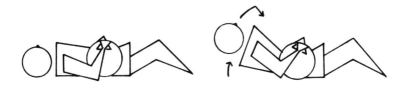

position: Lying on back, knees bent, hands crossed over abdominal area.

action: Breathe in deeply. As you exhale, raise your head forward off the floor. Support the abdominal muscles and pull them in towards the center with your crossed hands or arms. Return slowly to horizontal position.

Raising only the head and shoulders exercises the recti muscles specifically.

Do as many as 50 of these per day to quickly repair recti separation. Until the gap is closed, avoid exercises which rotate the trunk, twist the hips, or bend the body to one side. After healing, check periodically for recti separation.

Once there is no recti separation, or a separation of only 1-2 fingers, then standard curl-ups can be done.

Standard Abdominal Curl-ups

position: Lying on back, knees bent, hands cupping the back of your head.

action: Press lower back against the floor. Inhale deeply. Upon exhaling, raise head and shoulders off the floor (reaching a 40° angle) and hold for 3 seconds. You should look toward the ceiling, maintaining a space about the size of a grapefruit between your chin and chest. Slowly return to starting position. Repeat 30-50 times a day, starting gradually at 10 times a day and building up toward a goal of 50.

PELVIC FLOOR

The muscles of the pelvic floor have been referred to as the center of a woman's muscular anatomy. These muscles are critical to a woman's current and future health.[6]

The muscles of the pelvic floor support the pelvic organs (bladder, uterus, and intestines) and control the perineal openings (urethra, vagina, and rectum). They form a figure-8 as they loop around the urethral and vaginal opening in front and the anal opening in the back. The middle section between the anus and the vagina (where the figure-8 crosses) is called the perineum.

The tone and elasticity of the pelvic floor enables voluntary control of elimination and prevents involuntary relaxation of the sphincters (perineal openings). Pelvic floor muscles provide resistance to the pressures of laughing, coughing, sneezing, lifting, pushing, and elimination.

Weakness caused by the pressures of pregnancy, the strain of childbirth, and the simple force of gravity can cause the pelvic muscle floor to sag. Excessive sagging can result in serious structural changes and impairment of function. Loss of urinary control is the most characteristic symptom of the laxity of pelvic floor muscles. Stress incontinence occurs in various degrees from incontinence only with severe stress, such as sneezing or running, to incontinence as a result of moderate stress such as walking up and down stairs or simply standing

upright. Protective undergarments may even be necessary. Other symptoms resulting from sagging pelvic floor
muscles include a heavy achy feeling, inability to retain
a tampon, and decreased pleasure during marital relations.

Problems with pelvic floor function become more serious with succeeding pregnancies, increasing age, and
decreasing hormones after menopause. It is, therefore,
essential to strengthen and repair the pelvic floor muscles during and between pregnancies. Exercise is the
treatment of choice for sagging pelvic muscles. However,
if there is severe organ prolapse (the uterus protrudes
through the vaginal outlet), surgery may be required.

KEGEL EXERCISES

Kegel exercises involve tightening and releasing the
pelvic floor muscles.

You can test yourself to be sure you are exercising the
right muscles by stopping and starting urination (with
no dribbling). Avoid doing this first thing in the morning
or when you have a full bladder. Also, do not attempt
this test when you have a urinary tract infection.

Generally speaking, kegels can be done anytime, anywhere. Only you know that you are doing them. You can
do them when sitting, standing or lying down.

▸ Exhale while drawing up the perineal muscles (feel
them tighten). Hold for two to three seconds and release.

▸ Progress to doing 5 kegels in a row, holding for 5
seconds each.

▸ A creative alternative is to imagine you are riding in
an elevator. Progressively tighten the perineal muscles
as you "go up" a few floors, then gradually relax as you
descend to ground level. Gently exhale through pursed
lips throughout the exercise.

▸ For women with pelvic floor problems, two hundred
kegels a day are the recommended therapeutic solution.

▸ For the average woman, fifty kegels a day in sets of
five are recommended.

❧ ❧ ❧ ❧ ❧

Additional   Here are two additional exercises that you may en-
Exercises   joy doing.

According to Elizabeth Noble, squatting offers many
advantages for childbirth and is necessary for good body
mechanics in such actions as lifting without stooping.

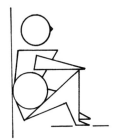

Exercise 3: Prenatal Squatting

With your back against the wall, hold
onto a firm support, such as a chair or a
doorway. Feet should be flat on the
floor and wide apart. Lower your body
slowly to squatting position. Hold for 3-5
seconds. Repeat 5 times.

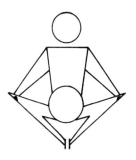

Exercise 4: Prenatal Tailor Sitting

Sit with your back straight and the soles
of your feet together. Hands are under
the knees. [*Do not* do this exercise if you
experience any pain in the area of the
pubic bones, as separation of this fibrous union may be present.] Press both
your knees toward the floor while providing resistance with your hands. Hold for
3 seconds and release. Repeat 5-10
times.

NOTES

1. Rambam, *Hilchos De'os* 4:2, 6, 13, 14.
2. N. Hacker, J. Moore, *Essentials of Obstetrics and Gynecology* (Philadelphia: W. B. Saunders & Co., 1986), p. 58.
3. *Health Almanac, U.S. News and World Report* (1990), p. 31.
4. Rambam, *Hilchos De'os* 4:2.
5. Elizabeth Noble, *Essential Exercises for the Childbearing Year* (Boston: Houghton Mifflin Company, 1988).
6. Ibid.

PART TWO:

The Perinatal Phase

10 | Approaching the Due Date

More powerful is the preparation for a
mitzvah than the actual performance of
the mitzvah itself.
SEFAS EMES, PARASHAS HA'AZINU

When a woman reaches her third trimester, she starts to realize that the actual birth is not so far away. This can be a shocking, yet exciting, jolt into reality. Many mothers find that this is the time to start to learn (or brush up on) childbirth and nursing techniques.

Preparation for Childbirth   Childbirth preparation classes begin around the 28th week of pregnancy. They are given either as a service of the hospital or privately by certified instructors. A good childbirth course offers a balanced approach, presenting various options. It is important to make sure that the person teaching the course is a qualified, professional childbirth educator.

Childbirth preparation classes are generally very encouraging. It is always comforting to know that you are not the only woman going through this experience. Scientific studies have demonstrated a dramatic difference in the experiences of women who are knowledgeable and prepared for childbirth and women who are not. Positive and realistic expectations for pregnancy and childbirth create a relaxed atmosphere, which can subsequently lead to a quicker delivery.

A study of 500 patients compared women who had prepared for childbirth using the Lamaze method to women who did not attend childbirth preparation classes. The trained women had one-fourth the number of cesarean sections, one-fifth the amount of fetal distress, and one-third the number of postpartum infections.[1]

Dr. Grantly Dick-Read developed the earliest theories of what we today call "natural childbirth." He believed that eliminating fear through proper instruction could reduce the pain of childbirth. He did, however, advocate the use of pain medication when necessary.

The Lamaze method, which was popularized by the French physician Ferdinand Lamaze, is based on theories of behavioral conditioning. The woman practices an automatic stimulus-response behavior to achieve relaxation. By focusing on controlled breathing, she can be distracted from pain and use this tool to cooperate with the medical staff to make her delivery easier.

The Bradley method of prepared childbirth specifically emphasizes the husband's contribution in the form of coaching and encouraging his wife during labor and delivery.

Childbirth: A Team Approach

Natural childbirth techniques do not just focus on easing the pain of contractions. Offering encouragement during the relaxation periods between contractions is a very important factor. Although providing a cold drink or assistance is helpful, what really encourages a woman and gives her the feeling of strength and security is warm and loving emotional support. Feeling secure can also render practical medical benefits.

Having a coach with you during labor can insure that you will be as relaxed as possible. It is so reassuring to know that there is someone there for you, in addition to the medical staff (as helpful as they may be). Your coach will help you maintain the proper breathing patterns, distract you from any discomfort, and be a partner in any care decisions that may need to be made during labor and delivery.

Choosing the right coach is an individual decision. One woman might want her husband with her, while another may prefer her mother or sister. Yet another might choose a good friend or hire a professional coach. Each couple should take all the factors into consideration when making their decision (see Chapter 13 on Labor and Delivery).

In addition to halachic considerations (for Halachah about husbands in the labor room, see pp. 145-46), you and your husband should consider your own personal relationship. Moreover, some husbands may be queasy or feel uncomfortable when faced with medical realities, and many find it difficult to watch their wives suffering any discomfort. These husbands may gladly relinquish their coaching roles to others. On the other hand, many husbands feel they can be of real assistance to their wives and after the birth feel tremendously exhilarated at having participated in this important family event.

Whomever you choose to share your birth experience, he or she can make a big difference.

The idea of coaching and encouraging during labor and delivery has roots in ancient Jewish history. The Torah tells us that the names of the two Jewish midwives who risked their lives to deliver the Jewish babies in Egypt were Shifrah and Puah. The *Midrash* explains that the name Shifrah is derived from the Hebrew word *leshaper*, meaning "to improve" or "make better". This refers to Shifrah's concern and care for the newborn infants. Puah's name derives from the Hebrew word meaning "cry out." The *Matnas Kehunah* says that she would speak to the Jewish women, and as a result they would give birth without pain.

According to *Chazal*, Puah was Miriam. She was a very wise and considerate midwife who understood that the attitude of the mother could have a tremendous effect on her perception of pain. Therefore, Miriam would encourage and help each woman so that she would experience a less painful birth.[2]

Although men are truly interested in their wives' welfare, most are embarrassed by the subject matter covered in these classes. Since the entire subject is so personal and feminine, it is not appropriate for the husband to attend the course. Many women feel that it is immodest, and in fact difficult, to discuss such personal topics in front of another woman's husband. Certainly, it is halachically forbidden for women to be exercising or practicing breathing techniques while lying on the floor in a mixed group. Therefore, only women should attend childbirth courses.

Childbirth Classes and Husbands

A possible option for involving the husband is to schedule one individual session between the instructor and the couple. This private meeting can focus on any personal questions or problems the couple may have. Pertinent information can be shared after each class, and breathing exercises can be practiced privately, in the more modest and comfortable setting of the home. Thus, without attending a mixed class, the husband can learn everything necessary to play an active role in the couple's childbirth experience.

How do we understand the concept of natural childbirth? It certainly does not mean going back to the primitive conditions of a hundred years ago, when it was "natural" for a woman to receive no prenatal care and to deliver her baby without qualified medical supervision. It is worthwhile to recall that this type of childbirth was accompanied by high maternal and infant mortality.

What Is Natural Childbirth?

Home delivery, where anything can happen and the appropriate emergency facilities are not available, is a potentially life-threatening situation. By choosing to give birth at home, a woman could be putting herself and her baby in serious danger. Since the risks are so great, the *halachah* of *piku'ach nefesh,* and not personal priorities, must be taken into consideration before opting for a home birth.

In the Western world today, natural childbirth takes place in the hospital, without drugs or medical assistance and many women hope that their labor and delivery will be uncomplicated and free from hospital interference. However, as we will see throughout this chapter, medical intervention is sometimes required during labor and delivery. Whether medical intervention was necessary or not, the most positive childbirth experience is the method of childbirth most conducive to the health of both mother and baby — which is "naturally" the right thing to do.

Pain in Childbirth   Each woman has her own way of handling stress, happiness, frustration, and affection. She also has her own threshold and level of tolerance for pain. Some women may never have been put to the test, and labor may be the first opportunity for them to discover their personal tolerance for pain.

It is customary in childbirth classes to view a documentary featuring a delivery where breathing techniques are employed. In this documentary, the woman generally smiles throughout childbirth. How wonderful! But most women will affirm that, in reality, childbirth is a physically painful experience.

A positive attitude, however, does significantly improve the situation. Realizing that there is a rational, understandable reason for the pain, knowing that the pain is self-limiting and not indefinite, and, finally, looking forward to the special reward at the end of the experience, all contribute to an easier delivery. Knowledge, preparation and support can help you face the childbirth experience with calm and control.

You must also accept that there are many things which are not in your control, such as the strength of the contractions, your own strength, and possible complications. You are not the woman in the documentary, and you are not just like your next-door neighbor. You will be undergoing a personal, and highly individual experience. Therefore, you should not make a firm decision about pain relief before the onset of labor.

Since pain is subjective, it is impossible to give an accurate description of what you will feel during labor and delivery. However, there are general guidelines as to what you may expect. **Dealing with Pain**

Uterine contractions sweep from the back toward the stomach, though they are concentrated mainly in the abdominal area. The pain is intermittent: a tightening, lasting 45-60 seconds, at intervals ranging from every 20 minutes to 2-3 minutes apart. Each contraction begins with a minimal amount of discomfort, gradually increases in intensity, reaches its peak, and then declines in severity.

As the baby descends into the birth canal, cramp-like pains and pressure are felt in the lower abdomen and pelvis. Some women suffer from a concentration of pain in the lower back during labor, commonly known as BACK LABOR. This occurs when the baby's descending head exerts pressure on the nerve endings of the lower back.

Finally, as the baby descends further through the birth canal, an intense burning and pulling sensation may be felt.

The following section reviews various options of pain relief to provide the information you will need to make an intelligent and rational decision.

As the discomfort of labor intensifies, you will need to employ all the resources you have to cope with the discomfort and pain of the uterine contractions **Breathing Techniques**
and the dilating cervix. Breathing techniques which foster relaxation are extremely useful by themselves and can supplement any pain medication or epidural anesthesia you may receive.

Proper breathing throughout labor is important both

for the mother and the soon-to-be-born baby. By inhaling and exhaling efficiently, you will make maximum use of your strength and also promote an overall good feeling. Your baby, whose blood and oxygen supply is constricted with every contraction, will also benefit from the extra oxygen you generate throughout your body and his.

We all know that taking a deep breath can help us relax and gather strength whenever we are in a tense situation. The same holds true with breathing techniques, which help us relax and enable us to distance ourselves from the pain we are experiencing.

In order to practice these techniques, you will need a watch with a second hand to help you visualize a 60-second contraction which peaks in strength in the middle and then gradually diminishes in strength. The recommended position for practice is sitting or reclining.

The basic rules of proper breathing during and between contractions are:

❧ Always inhale through your nose and exhale through your mouth.

❧ When exhaling, purse your lips together in an "O" shape to direct your breath outward in a controlled manner.

❧ If your nose is congested, inhale through your mouth, placing your tongue behind your top teeth to prevent a dry mouth.

Practicing breathing techniques will help you avoid problems which improper breathing may cause. For example, breathing too rapidly can cause hyperventilation. Signs of hyperventilation include: tingling of the hands, lightheadedness, and dizziness. If you notice these symptoms, simply cup your hands over your nose and mouth, and breathe slowly and deeply. This will restore the proper carbon dioxide-oxygen balance in the body. If your mouth gets too dry, frequent sips of water or crushed ice will help.

There are three breathing techniques that will be helpful to you: deep-chest breathing, shallow-chest breathing, and rapid-chest breathing.

DEEP-CHEST BREATHING is employed during latent phase contractions (early, mild labor) or medical procedures. It induces relaxation and can lower a racing pulse rate. Some women are successful with this breathing level throughout their entire labor.

Inhale for 2 counts (seconds) and exhale slowly over 4 counts. You will average about 10 of these deep-chest breaths to 1 contraction.

SHALLOW-CHEST BREATHING is quite easy and helps you cope with the increasingly intense contractions of the active phase (intermediate, more intense labor).

Inhale, pause briefly, and exhale evenly over 2 counts. You will average about 25-30 shallow chest breaths to one contraction.

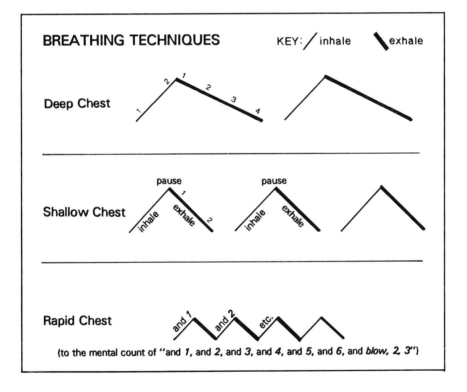

RAPID-CHEST BREATHING can help you maintain control during the transition segment (the most frequent and intense labor pains) and will also provide the oxygen you and your baby need.

After six rapid breaths (one sequence) exhale slowly for a count of three. You will average between 8 and 10 rapid-chest sequences during one contraction.

Breathe normally between contractions.

Practicing breathing techniques will build up the endurance that you need during labor. When you first begin to practice, you will feel tired and lightheaded, like an athlete preparing for a marathon. However, as you build up your endurance, the breathing levels will become an easy and natural routine. It is recommended that you practice about four times a week during the eighth and ninth month of pregnancy.

Your husband, a friend, or a labor coach will be an integral part of your success. He or she can remind you of the "dos and don'ts" and help you pace your breathing by breathing right along with you. The labor pains can disrupt your ability to follow the breathing patterns that will help relieve some of the discomfort, while your coach, who is not experiencing the pain, is able to maintain the breathing rhythm for you.

In addition to mastering the relaxation breathing techniques, there are other resources you can use to feel as comfortable as possible during labor. Learn not to tense up with the contractions, but to flow with them. The goal is not to fight the contractions but to work with them in order to conserve your energy for the second stage of labor.

EFFLUERAGE is gentle, circular stroking of the abdomen with your fingertips. It can relax you and also distract you from labor discomfort.

VISUALIZATION can also help. As the contraction intensifies, imagine yourself climbing a mountain to its peak and coming back down as the pain recedes. Davening or saying *Tehillim* can also build your inner strength. Some women distract themselves by listening to music. Placing a cool, wet cloth over your forehead and face is extremely refreshing. Whatever helps you to achieve maximum relaxation is acceptable.

Pain from back labor can be sharp and intense. One way to minimize the discomfort is by positioning yourself on all fours. This will shift the weight of the baby away from the affected nerve endings, but it is only effective for a short time.

Another way to relieve pain from back labor is to exert counter-pressure. You, or the person who has come to be with you during labor, may gently massage or push on the sacral (lower back) area with a hand, some tennis balls inserted into a sock, or even a rolling pin. This will also reduce the pressure on the nerve endings.

Anesthesia

Alternatively, pain relief may be obtained in the form of medical intervention. The pain of uterine contractions and childbirth can be effectively lessened or even eliminated with the use of anesthesia. The four most common forms of obstetrical anesthesia are demerol, pudendal block, epidural anesthesia, and penthrane gas.

DEMEROL: The analgesic, demerol (pethidine/dolestine), can be given by intramuscular injection (I.M.) or intravenously (I.V.) in doses of 50 mg., 75 mg., or 100 mg. It takes the edge off the contractions by reducing the intensity of pain. Since demerol may cause drowsiness, it is especially helpful for a woman who is tense and overtired, allowing her to relax and get the rest she so desperately needs. Another benefit of demerol is that it can cause the cervix to soften and dilate more quickly.

When given in the buttocks (I.M.), demerol takes effect in about 15 minutes, peaking at about 45 minutes and lasting for about 3-4 hours. When given intravenously, it is diluted in saline or glucose and administered like any other I.V. solution. It becomes effective within 5 minutes, peaks at around 20 minutes, and lasts from 2-3 hours.

Demerol may be given once contractions are regular and labor has reached the active phase. If labor is long and intense and delivery is not imminent, a second dose can be given four hours after the first dose.

The baby's heartbeat will register a sleeping pattern for the first half hour after demerol is administered. If there is any sign of fetal distress, demerol will not be given, since it can further depress central nervous system responses and heart rate. If administered too close to delivery, the baby may be born drowsy and hypotonic (with dulled reflexes). An antidote — Narcan — is then administered to rapidly "perk up" the baby's responses. Incidents of babies born hypotonic as a result of the demerol anesthetic are atypical, however, as the medical staff takes great care to give demerol at the correct time during labor.

Some women are uncomfortable with the lack of control they feel under the influence of demerol. Also, the woman is generally confined to bed for at least 3 hours after receiving this drug, because it can bring on nausea, vomiting and dizziness.

PUDENDAL BLOCK: A pudendal block is a means of anesthetizing the cervix and the perineum. Lidocaine is administered with a long needle through the vagina to the pudendal nerve. The entire perineal area becomes numb, reducing pain during episiotomy (a surgical incision to widen the vaginal opening) and delivery. A stinging sensation may be felt as the lidocaine is injected.

EPIDURAL ANESTHESIA: Many women refer to epidural anesthesia as a miracle. With it, the entire lower half of the body is relieved of pain. Mild pressure can still be felt, and the woman can push when necessary.

This procedure is performed either while the woman lies on her left side curled up like a cat, or while sitting up. An anesthesiologist injects lidocaine as a local anesthetic to the lower back. A needle is inserted between two of the lumbar vertebrae and then removed, leaving a fine thread-like catheter into which further anesthesia is injected.

That's it! The procedure is similar to a simple injection, and your husband or coach can stay with you the entire time.

After the anesthesia is injected, the woman remains on her back for 15 minutes to allow the anesthesia to distribute itself evenly. Then she can once again turn to her left side.

No pain is felt during labor and delivery by 95% of the women who are given epidural anesthesia. An epidural also relaxes the pelvic floor, which can hasten dilation. The mother is awake and aware throughout, and feels neither the episiotomy nor the suturing. As soon as pain is felt, additional anesthesia can be injected into the catheter.

Another advantage is that once an epidural is in place, the woman can proceed directly to cesarean section if necessary, requiring no further anesthesia. For this reason many doctors will prefer using epidural anesthesia for a woman who is having regular labor and delivery after a previous cesarean section.

An epidural is considered safer than general anesthesia. Also, because it is administered into the endural space before the spinal canal, an epidural does not produce the headaches and other complications caused by spinal anesthesia.

As long as the mother's blood pressure is maintained, there are no side effects for the baby. She will be connected to an I.V. at all times to receive fluids to keep her blood pressure from falling, which can lower the fetal heart rate. Oxygen may also be administered. With the lower half of her body numb, the mother will find it difficult to move. Therefore, she must remain in bed. Pushing may be difficult for some women, as the urge to push is greatly diminished.

Failure of an epidural to relieve pain is rare. It will occur only in five percent of cases and is usually attributable to back problems (structural defects), obesity, or an uncooperative patient.

PENTHRANE GAS: Sometimes penthrane gas (methoxy-flurane) is employed as an inhalation anesthetic. Although it is not used frequently, many delivery rooms offer penthrane for a short period of time during the transition segment of labor, before the mother begins to push.

Penthrane gas is administered through a gas mask, which a woman holds herself. When she breathes deeply, a sleepy, floating feeling is induced which takes the "bite" off a difficult contraction. The mask is removed between contractions.

Penthrane has a short-term effect, and it is rapidly metabolized in the body. It can cause respiratory depression in both the mother and the fetus, and can also increase intrapartum and postpartum blood loss.

IN SUMMARY: Of course, it is best to avoid medication during labor and delivery. However, this is not possible in all cases. When medication is necessary, proper breathing and relaxation techniques can enhance its effectiveness. The combination of medical and natural methods of childbirth thus results in the greatest comfort and safety for mother and child.

Complications before the Due Date   Although complications can occur before the due date, ninety percent of all pregnancies progress normally until delivery. Pre-term delivery (before the 37th week of pregnancy) is the most common of all possible complications.

A primary symptom of impending pre-term delivery is premature contractions. Even before the contractions are felt, a woman may notice increased vaginal discharge, pressure in the lower back, or cramps similar to those felt during menstruation. These symptoms often precede the development of premature contractions and should be brought to the attention of the obstetrician.

During the third trimester, it is normal for a woman to feel her uterus contract and relax at irregular intervals throughout the day. These "false" contractions, commonly known as "Braxton Hicks," occur more frequently as the due date approaches. Braxton Hicks are not painful, may last from 45 seconds to 2 minutes, and do not cause cervical dilation. (See Chapter 13 on Labor and Delivery for a detailed comparison of true vs. false labor.)

Contractions before the 37th week which occur at regular intervals with accompanying back pain and pressure in the pelvic region are a cause for concern.

POSSIBLE CAUSES OF PREMATURE CONTRACTIONS

Illness or infection can often be a cause of pre-term labor. Therefore, a pregnant woman with an elevated temperature (above 99°F/37.3°C) should notify her physician. She will probably be advised to take acetaminophen (Tylenol/Acamol) to bring the temperature down.

Cervical incompetence. Sometimes structural defects in the uterus or cervix prevent a woman from reaching full term. Cervical incompetence is an abnormality in which the cervix cannot remain closed and retain the fetus for the entire duration of the pregnancy. It may cause a rapid premature delivery, which may occur even without contractions. The diagnosis of an incompetent cervix is usually made only after a previous premature delivery. The treatment of choice is cervical cerclage. This procedure involves the suturing of the cervix, and is performed under general anesthesia at approximately week 14. Sutures are removed by week 37 or 38, or with the onset of labor.

Premature rupture of amniotic membranes (PROM) is another cause of pre-term labor. If the waters break before the 37th week, immediate hospitalization and constant supervision is required. When the waters break, the mucous plug — which served to "seal off" the uterus and its contents from possible infection — is lost. Therefore, the expectant mother's temperature and white blood cell count are continually monitored for any elevation. If contractions do not begin spontaneously, the medical staff may attempt to delay delivery as long as there are no signs of infection, cervical dilation, and the well-being of the fetus is assured.

Pre-term labor can also be caused by uterine malformations, multiple pregnancy (twins, triplets, etc.) or fetal abnormalities. However, the major cause of premature contractions is dehydration. Although a pregnant woman may feel she is drinking adequately, her body may still be lacking in the fluids it needs.

PREVENTING PRE-TERM LABOR

A woman having premature contractions at intervals of every 20 minutes or less should take steps to prevent the contractions from becoming more severe. Absolute rest for one hour and drinking at least one quart (1 liter) of fluids should stop the contractions. If they do not stop, then she must go to a hospital for more intensive medical care, which will include the intravenous administration of fluids. If contractions are treated before cervical dilation begins, intravenous fluids (1-2 liters of saline or 5% glucose) should be enough to stem further progression of contractions without medication.

When premature contractions cannot be stopped with fluids alone, a uterine relaxant (ritodrine/yutopar) is administered either intravenously or orally, requiring hospitalization. Upon discharge from the hospital, a woman may continue with this medication until the ninth month.

If advancing cervical dilation or deterioration in either the mother's or the baby's condition dictates pre-term birth, the mother may be given glucocorticoid (dexamethasone) injections to promote lung maturity in the fetus. These injections can save the baby's life by preventing the most common complication of pre-term infants — respiratory difficulties.

PREMATURE DELIVERY

In order to prevent trauma for the baby, a cesarean section may be performed. If the delivery is vaginal, the amniotic membranes will not be broken until immediately before delivery. By waiting until just before delivery, there will be less pressure on the baby's skull.

Premature delivery can be traumatic for the parents and entails a long recuperative process for the newborn. When caring for a pre-term infant, it is especially important to: maintain warmth, give oxygen and respiratory therapy when necessary, avoid infection, and provide appropriate nutrition. These services are provided in a special neonatal intensive care unit.

While breast milk is the food of choice, not all preemies are able to suck. Babies born before the 34th week do not have a mature sucking reflex. Until the baby learns to suck, he will be fed by means of a feeding tube inserted through the nose and leading into the stomach.

The new mother will want to provide her own breast milk for her baby, which also enables her to maintain her own milk supply. She should therefore make use of an electric breast pump, which is usually available at each neonatal facility. As the baby grows, the mother will be able to nurse him directly.

New parents are encouraged to touch and even hold their premature newborn. Thus a special bond is developed, which helps both parents and baby get over this especially difficult period.

Warning Signs for Immediate Attention

During the third trimester of pregnancy, a woman must be especially aware of the signals her body is transmitting. It is useful for every expectant mother to understand the implications of certain symptoms which require immediate medical attention.

Bleeding: A tablespoon or more of bright red blood is a signal of possible hemorrhage and the separation of the placenta from the uterus.

Severe abdominal pain: Another possible warning of hemorrhage is a constant, sharp abdominal pain, which does not allow the woman to stand up straight. Bleeding may be obvious or concealed in the uterus.

Change in the pattern of fetal movements: Towards the end of pregnancy, the baby is encumbered by being cramped into a very small area. In addition, the placenta's functioning capacity is naturally reduced as it begins to age and form fibrous deposits. Placental aging combined with umbilical cord problems can also seriously hinder fetal movement. Despite these considerations, the mother should relate to any change from the routine pattern of fetal movements as an emergency requiring medical evaluation and fetal monitoring. If she feels that fetal movements have lessened or stopped altogether, she should consult her physician immediately. During pregnancy, it is incumbent upon each woman to become familiar enough with the characteristics of her baby's movements to detect a significant change.

Assessment of Fetal Movements

It is natural for an expectant mother to want to know at all times that her baby is active and healthy. She can easily assess this by paying extra attention to her baby's movements.

Some babies are more active than others, but usually within two hours of your last meal you should be able to feel your baby being quite active. If not, lie on your left side in a quiet room — you should feel at least 4-6 fetal movements in half an hour. If after one hour you feel no fetal movements, or fewer fetal movements than normally felt, phone your doctor or go directly to the hospital, where a fetal monitor will be used to assess the baby's well-being.

Pack a Bag

During your ninth month, as your due date approaches, it is time to pack a bag with all the things you will need for your hospital stay. Being prepared will save you from a last-minute rush and from forgetting items which you will want to have with you.

WHAT TO BRING TO THE HOSPITAL:

An envelope containing: medical records, ultrasound
results, hospital registration form, insurance documents, prepared cards detailing personal information*
Siddur and *Tehillim*
reading material, paper and pen
towel, washcloth
nightgown, robe
6-8 pairs of disposable underwear (or old underwear
which you won't mind discarding)
slippers
socks/stockings
extra head coverings
nursing bra, nursing pads, at least 2 safety pins
Vitamin E oil
liquid soap, shampoo
toothbrush, toothpaste
pocket money
phone directory, change/telephone card/phone tokens
THIS BOOK!

*See Chapter 12 on Going to the Hospital on Shabbos.

NOTES

1. M.J. Hyghly, "Maternal and Fetal Outcome of Lamaze Prepared
   Patients, *Obstetrics and Gynecology* 51:653, 1978.
2. *Koheles Rabbah* 7; *see* Hebrew appendix.

11 | Insuring a Safe Birth: A Torah Perspective

Treat His will as if it were your own will,
so that He will treat your will as if
it were His will.

PIRKEI AVOS 2:4

Different women experience a variety of emotions when relating to childbirth. The primary concern of all women, however, is to have a safe birth. Women will often go to great lengths to insure a safe birth: engaging a private doctor or midwife, selecting the best hospital, and so forth. Some women rely on *segulos* (religious luck charms or amulets), which they bring along to the delivery room. And certainly, all women pray.

The advice of *Chazal* as to how to insure a safe birth is also relevant to the essence of Jewish womanhood. The Mishnah tells us that there is potential danger in childbirth for a woman who is careless with three mitzvos: *niddah* (the Laws of Family Purity), *challah* (separating a portion of dough to give to the *kohen*), and lighting the Shabbos candles.[1]

The Talmud asks why punishment for these transgressions is given at childbirth as opposed to any other time. Common to the many answers is the notion that at a time of potential danger *Hakadosh Baruch Hu* exacts payment for a sin.

The Talmud then asks when men are tested. In other words, when do men make payment for their sins? The Talmud answers that men are judged (or punished) for their sins when they pass over a bridge or experience any extreme danger.[2]

It is interesting to note that women are not judged during every dangerous encounter, as men are. Their crucible occurs at one very specific hour of danger: childbirth. The question is obvious — Why is childbirth precisely the instant when a woman is tested?

Another question arises when considering the differences in punishment between men and women. Whereas restitution is exacted from men for any sin at all times of danger, women are punished for transgressions against the specific Laws of Family Purity, taking a portion of the challah, and candlelighting (and only during childbirth). After all, women are obligated to keep all the mitzvos just as men are (with the exception of positive commandments which are related to time). What is the specific relationship of these three commandments to childbirth?

The Talmud tells us that woman was created only to have children and to be beautiful.[3] Could this be the only purpose of woman? Surely even the most adamant male chauvinist would consider this view extreme. What, then, is the real meaning of this statement?

The Uniqueness of Woman

Creation came into being level by level, with each new level being greater than the previous one. Man is the ultimate level and incorporates a Divine aspect. And yet, another creation came into being after man — woman. The Talmud concerns itself with the philosophical question: What did woman add to the world? What attributes did Hashem endow woman with that man did not already possess? The answer is: Woman's unique contributions to the world are her ability to bear and raise children, and her beauty. In other words, a woman possesses the same attributes as man, but with an addition — the ability to bring children and beauty into the world.

Beauty does not refer solely to the woman's personal beauty, but also to an appreciation for beauty in general — what we call "the woman's touch." The feminine talents of decorating a home, arranging flowers, coordinating colors, selecting clothing, and so forth, enhance the aesthetic loveliness of the world.

The ability of a woman to bear a child is what sets her apart from man physically. Her different physiological makeup is specifically suited for childbirth. Therefore, childbirth is not merely a biological act but an expression of her special merit, the essence of her partnership with Hashem. She brings life into the world and enables mankind to continue.

Woman: Three Components, Three Mitzvos

Everything in the world is made up of three components: substance, form and purpose.[4] A table, for example, is made from the substance of wood, its form is four legs and a board, and its purpose is for objects to be placed upon it.

The three pilgrim holidays also correspond to these three components. Pesach represents the Jewish People becoming a nation, which is the substance. Shavuos, when we received the Torah, represents the form to which the Jewish People must adhere — the Torah way of life. And Sukkos represents our purpose: to sit in a "sacred" house — *Olam Ha-ba* — and in this world, to be a "kingdom of priests and a holy nation."

A woman's femininity may also be broken down into these three components. Her body is the substance, her life style the form, and her purpose is the ideal fulfillment of her combined substance and form.

Three mitzvos correspond to the three components of womanhood, bringing each to the level of the sacred. They are: family purity, separating *challah*, and lighting the Shabbos candles. The Laws of Family Purity deal with the woman's body. They add sanctity to the physi-

ological process which is the "substance" of her femininity. By observing the *niddah* laws, she elevates her body
to holiness and purity.

The act of separating *challah* is symbolic of the lifestyle of *chesed* (lovingkindness) which should personify
the woman. The *challah* was once given to the *kohen*,
but the act is more than merely a gift of monetary value.
First the woman must knead the dough, and invest a
part of herself in it. When she gives the *challah*, she is
giving of her own hard work, an even greater gift than
one of money. In this way she sanctifies her feminine
"form."

When the Jewish People were wandering in the desert, it was the women who excelled in sanctifying themselves in these two respects (substance and form). When
the spies spoke about Eretz Yisrael in a derogatory manner, it was the men who responded with weeping. The
women did not participate in that sin, as we learn from
the daughters of Tzelofchad, who requested a portion in
Eretz Yisrael (*Bemidbar* 27).

The *Kli Yakar* analyzes the difference between the
men and the women of that generation. One factor which
distanced the men from the Land was the fact that Eretz
Yisrael would not tolerate immoral behavior. Since some
of the men felt that they could not withstand temptation,
they chose to return to Egypt, a land so corrupt that it
would easily tolerate immoral behavior. On the other
hand, the women were essentially very modest and
strove to sanctify themselves. They therefore related to
Eretz Yisrael as the perfect place in which to refine their
modesty and sanctity.

Another factor to which the men had difficulty relating was the strictness of those laws applying only in
Eretz Yisrael, which demand of every citizen that he forfeit significant portions of his produce. *Terumos* and
ma'asros go to the *kohen* and the *levi. Leket* and
shichechah go to the poor. The men felt that it was futile
to work so hard in order to give so much to others. They

were not happy to give the *tzedakah* which Eretz Yisrael required. Therefore, they preferred to stay out of Israel. The women, on the other hand, loved the mitzvos of *chesed*, especially the mitzvah of separating *challah.* They desired to live in Eretz Yisrael, a place where it was more conducive to give.

The third mitzvah, lighting Shabbos candles, represents the "purpose" of the Jewish woman. The source of the Jewish nation's strength has always been its home life, through which every Jew becomes deeply rooted in his heritage. The woman is the *akeres ha-bayis*, the foundation of the home. She is responsible for shaping and molding her children into God-fearing Jews. Lighting candles is more than just producing a physical illumination: "*Ner mitzvah v'Torah or* — The mitzvah is like a candle and the Torah is light." Lighting the candles on *erev Shabbos* symbolizes the woman's responsibility to light up her home with Torah and ethical values, thereby achieving her essential purpose.

Thus, fulfilling the Laws of Family Purity is the sanctification of the physical aspect of a woman's femininity, separating *challah* represents the lifestyle of giving, and lighting Shabbos candles is symbolic of the purpose of the woman — to light up her home with Torah.

In view of the above, we can understand why carelessness in these mitzvos is remembered at the time of childbirth. Since childbirth is unique to the woman and the paramount expression of her femininity, a defect in these three aspects — substance, form and purpose — negates her femininity so that she cannot withstand the judgment at the very moment she is performing her essential feminine function.

On the other hand, we have the ability to reverse this negative consequence and make childbirth a positive and holy experience by being careful in observing the Laws of Family Purity, separating *challah,* and lighting candles. In this way, we sanctify our bodies, lead a life of *chesed,* and illuminate our homes with Torah and ethics. Our femininity is thus realized through the ultimate spiritual expression.

During childbirth, womanhood's finest hour, we merit to join *Hakadosh Baruch Hu* as His partner in bringing new life into the world.

NOTES

1. *Mishnah Shabbos* 2:6.
2. *Shabbos* 32a.
3. *Kesubbos* 59b.
4. *See* Malbim, *Vayikra* 23:43.

12 | Going to the Hospital on Shabbos

*Override the laws of one Sabbath in order
to keep many other Sabbaths.*
YOMA 85b

A major concern for all religious women is the proper procedure involved in going to the hospital on Shabbos or *Yom Tov*. With careful preparation, you can minimize the need to overstep the bounds of Shabbos.[1]

As soon as you begin the ninth month, and certainly after your due date, you must accept that the possibility exists that you may have to go to the hospital on Shabbos. During the week, make local babysitting arrangements for your other young children so that you will not have to drive them anywhere on Shabbos. Before each Shabbos, prepare your house, car, and overnight bag so that everything will be ready if needed, and you will be able to keep your anxiety down to a minimum.

Preparing the House It is advisable to leave at least one light on in the house, in case you awaken with contractions during the night. Leave the telephone connected.

Preparing the Car If you will be going to the hospital in your own car, disconnect all unnecessary lights (door lights, trunk light, car alarm). Lights which are needed for safety, such as headlights, taillights, and brake lights, should obviously not be disconnected.

It is not required that you remove unnecessary items normally kept in the car, such as baby car seats, maps, etc.[2] However, if the hospital is outside the *techum Shabbos* (2,000 cubits or one mil, which is 1,028 yards outside the city limits), these items must be removed from the car (providing the car is within an *eruv*),[3] unless, of course, you feel there is no time to do so. (Preferably, these items should be removed before Shabbos.)

Preparing a Bag

As was already discussed, you should have a travel bag ready at all times during your ninth month. In addition to everything you need for your hospital stay, you should prepare a few cards with:

your name and address	your blood type
your father's name	name of health insurance
your husband's name	name of hospital
your social security/identification number	

It is not necessary to remove the *muktzeh* from the bag before Shabbos as long as the bag contains a non-*muktzeh* item which has greater importance than the *muktzeh* item (either greater monetary value or greater importance in its specific Shabbos function, e.g., food).[4]

Even when the hospital is outside the *techum Shabbos*, you may take whatever you feel you might want to have. (Your escort may take food along also, as long as the house/hospital is inside an *eruv*.[5])

If the hospital and/or your house is not within the *eruv*, the overnight bag cannot be taken. If your house is not within the *eruv* and the hospital is, the bag may be placed in the car before Shabbos, so that it can be taken on Shabbos.

If the hospital does not have an *eruv*, the bag cannot be taken; however, the cards with pertinent medical information may be carried *k'le'achar yad* — in a different manner than usual — or carried higher than ten *tefachim* (approximately 3 feet above the ground).[6] Discuss this with a Rav for further clarification.

Outside Eretz Yisrael, it is preferable not to bring the card, as there will probably be a non-Jew available to write down the necessary information. (Some hospitals in Israel also have non-Jewish personnel.)

Transportation to the Hospital   The best way to go to the hospital is by ambulance because an ambulance contains all the necessary equipment for an emergency delivery. The next best option is to go by taxi, since the taxi driver has a radio with which he can call for help in case of an emergency. The last choice is by private car driven by your husband, parent or neighbor.[7]

The decision should be determined the same way it would be during the week (provided that the decision is based on efficiency and safety and not on monetary considerations). If you would normally go by ambulance, then do so on Shabbos; if by car, then do so on Shabbos.

CALLING FOR A RIDE

It is preferable to make the telephone call with a *shinui* (changing the normal procedure — for example, knocking the phone off the hook instead of lifting it normally, and dialing with a fork instead of using your finger). Some *poskim* say that two people can take the phone off the hook together (*shenayim she'asuha*), or that you may even remove the receiver with two hands if there is no one else at home. Others do not rely on these last two methods.[8]

The conversation should be short and concise. However, you need not omit words; it is even permissible to say hello, goodbye, and thank you. Once the telephone connection is made, there is no prohibition on the number of relevant words spoken.[9]

If you telephoned and ordered an ambulance or taxi service, then you may replace the receiver, since the line needs to remain open for other emergency calls. You should try, though, to do it with a *shinui*. However, if the call was made to someone who no longer needs the use of his phone on Shabbos (such as a neighbor), then the receiver should not be replaced until after Shabbos.

CALLING THE DOCTOR

It is permissible to call your own doctor or midwife on Shabbos even though the hospital has a staff of mid-wives and other doctors. Use a *shinui* as with calling an ambulance. This is permissible because it is very important that the woman feel as secure and reassured as possible.[10]

CHOOSING AN AMBULANCE SERVICE

If you would normally call a non-Jewish ambulance service, then you may do so on Shabbos. If you would normally call a Jewish ambulance service because you feel more secure, or feel that the Jewish service is more reliable, then you should do so on Shabbos. It is not necessary to specifically call a non-Jewish service so as to minimize *chillul Shabbos*; the primary concern is for the mother to reach the hospital quickly and safely, and to feel as confident and as reassured as possible.[11]

PAYING THE TAXI DRIVER

It is forbidden to handle money on Shabbos. There-fore, you should ask the taxi driver if it will be all right to pay him after Shabbos and leave with him some form of collateral (a watch, identity card, license). If he does not agree to payment after Shabbos, it is permissible to pay him but not to take change. You can prepare the ap-proximate amount of the fare in advance and then either forfeit the change or ask the driver to hold it for you un-til after Shabbos. It is best to phone the taxi service be-fore Shabbos, and come to an agreement regarding price and payment.[12]

CHOOSING THE HOSPITAL

If a woman feels that in one hospital she will receive better care than in another one, and the better one is further, she may choose to go there.[13] (In Israel, this also applies if the woman will feel better in a hospital which is *shomer Shabbos*. Therefore, even if the medical care given is equal in either hospital, she may travel to the hospital which is further away but *shomer Shabbos*.)

WHEN TO GO TO THE HOSPITAL

A detailed discussion of how to determine when to go to the hospital under standard circumstances can be found in Chapter 13 on Labor and Delivery. However, it is important to note that on Shabbos, the *halachah* allows travel to the hospital as soon as the woman has regular contractions and feels the need to go.[14]

ESCORT

Many *poskim* say that if a woman feels more secure traveling with someone she trusts, then either her husband, sister, or mother, etc., may accompany her. However, some *poskim* feel that most women are capable of traveling to the hospital by themselves, confident that they will be in competent medical hands. Therefore, there is no reason for a husband to travel with his wife unless she is in great need of an escort.[15] Because every particular case should be determined individually, one should consult a Rav before the problem arises.

PARKING THE CAR

Once the driver has reached his destination he is forbidden to continue driving in order to look for a parking spot. He must stop the car immediately even if that means in an illegal parking spot. However, if the parking spot is a safety hazard (e.g., blocking the hospital driveway), then he may continue until he finds the closest spot that is not a safety hazard.[16]

TURNING OFF THE IGNITION

It is preferable to ask a non-Jew to turn the ignition off for you. If this is not feasible, then the driver may turn the ignition off, preferably with a *shinui*. However, if by turning the ignition off, electric lights will go off as well (e.g., the dashboard lights), then it may only be done by a non-Jew, unless leaving the car engine on will be a safety hazard. If so, then the ignition may be turned off by a Jew (preferably with a *shinui*).[17]

Consult your Rav about returning home on Shabbos in case of it being a false alarm.[18]

There are many *halachos* that apply to going to the hospital on Shabbos, whether for a birth or any medical emergency. Since it is impossible to illustrate every case, it is best for parents to be familiar with the basic *halachos* of *piku'ach nefesh* and Shabbos. These are some of the general guidelines:

A. When "time is of the essence," the only consideration is getting the mother to the labor room on time.

1. One should not rely on a non-Jew to do the *melachah* for him.

2. One should not ask a Rav what to do — he should just go.

B. If using a *shinui* when performing a *melachah* will not cause any delay, then it is preferable to do so, but if it causes a delay then the *melachah* should be done in its usual manner.

C. When there is less of a rush, override the laws of Shabbos in a manner which least causes a Shabbos transgression.

The following are some of the problem areas:

Carrying car keys.

Cars with electric windows.

Entrance to the hospital via an electric door.

Elevators.

Bringing kosher food to a hospital with only non-kosher food supplies when there is no *eruv*.

If these or other situations pose potential problems for you, discuss them with your Rav before the ninth month. The last few chapters of *Shemiras Shabbos K'hilchasah** by Rabbi J.J. Neuwirth and *The Comprehensive Guide to Medical Halachah** by Dr. Abraham S. Abraham deal with these *halachos* in a more comprehensive fashion. Also, see *Toras Ha-Yoledes** by Rabbi Yitzchak Zilberstein and Dr. Moshe Rothschild. However, even after studying these works, it is advisable to discuss the principles of *piku'ach nefesh* with your Rav.

If problems arise unexpectedly, use the guidelines listed above and your common sense to weigh the seriousness of Shabbos against the safety considerations.

*Available in English from Feldheim Publishers.

NOTES

1. *Mishnah Berurah* 330:1.
2. R. Moshe Sternbuch, comments on *Toras Ha-Yoledes*.
3. *Shemiras Shabbos K'hilchasah* 40:65; *see* Hebrew appendix.
4. *See* Hebrew appendix.
5. *Shemiras Shabbos K'hilchasah* 40, note 136; also heard from R. Mordechai Eliyahu.
6. *Mishnah Berurah* 301:123; *see Shemiras Shabbos K'hilchasah* 40:66; *see also* Hebrew appendix.
7. According to R. Mordechai Eliyahu; *see Toras Ha-Yoledes* 10.
8. *Shemiras Shabbos K'hilchasah* 32:40 allows *melachah* being done by two people; *see Tzitz Eliezer* vol. XVII, ch. 20, who tends toward forbidding it; *see also Responsa, Or l'Tzion* vol. II, p.255, which says that no *shinui* is required at all.
9. *Shemiras Shabbos K'hilchasah* 32:41.
10. *Tzitz Eliezer* vol. XIII, 55.
11. *Shulchan Aruch* 328:12; Taz 328:5; *see* Hebrew appendix.
12. *See Toras Ha-Yoledes* 23; *Shemiras Shabbos K'hilchasah* 32:55.
13. *Shemiras Shabbos K'hilchasah* 36:8.
14. *Mishnah Berurah* 330:9.
15. *See* Hebrew appendix.
16. *Shemiras Shabbos K'hilchasah* 40:57.
17. Ibid., 40:59,60.
18. *See Iggros Moshe* vol. IV, 80, and *see also Minchas Yitzchak* 8 and *Shemiras Shabbos K'hilchasah* 36:5.

13 | Labor and Delivery

He does immeasurable greatness and
countless wonders.
IYOV 9:9

'He does immeasurable greatness' —
refers to the fetus in his mother's womb;
'and countless wonders' — refers to the
moment of birth.
OSIYOS D'RABBI AKIVA, ALEF

Labor and delivery are the culmination of pregnancy. However, the tremendous emphasis placed on the "main event" seems paradoxical when compared to the comprehensive picture of pregnancy, childbirth, and postpartum care. Labor and delivery usually last less than 24 hours — a time span which is relatively insignificant when measured against nine months of pregnancy or a lifetime of child-rearing. Perhaps the reason for the "center stage" attention is the drama, the challenge, and the excitement of the experience, which is never the same at any two deliveries. Or perhaps the reason is simply that there is something very special about the start of life.

Labor is a process of physiological adjustment to facilitate the passage of the baby from the uterus to the world. Acquiring the tools to make labor and delivery a positive experience does not mean merely learning how to breathe and relax. Knowledge of the fundamentals and procedures of childbirth will enable you to take an active role in your care, reduce fear, and help you maintain control at a time when you are so vulnerable and dependent upon the care of others.

One of the most important messages we can keep in mind at this time is the teaching of the Gemara.[1] There it is written that *Hakadosh Baruch Hu* holds three keys, which He will not relinquish to a *shaliach* (messenger): the key of rain, the key of birth, and the key of *techiyas ha-meisim* (the resurrection of the dead). The commentary of *Tosafos* teaches that the keys of rain and *techiyas ha-meisim* can be given over to a *shaliach*. However, *Hakadosh Baruch Hu* has never relinquished the key to birth. There can be no greater reassurance or comfort than being secure in the knowledge that Hashem Himself is by your side, supervising the safety of mother and baby.

Terminology of Labor and Delivery The CERVIX is the gate through which the baby must pass in order to enter the birth canal (vagina). It is commonly referred to as the neck of the uterus and is located at the lowest part of the uterus. The cervix contains few muscle cells, but it does have an abundance of nerve endings, and therefore is a very sensitive area. In preparation for birth, uterine contractions cause the lower segment of the uterus to shorten, opening the cervix. Thus, observation of the cervix is an essential tool in assessing progress during labor.

The cervix must undergo two alterations in order for labor to progress to delivery: CERVICAL DILATION and CERVICAL EFFACEMENT.

Cervical dilation refers to the opening of the cervix. Dilation is measured in centimeters from 0 (closed cervix) to 10 cm. (fully open). There are hospitals that measure cervical dilation by fingers (1 finger = 2 cm.), and using this terminology, five fingers would mean complete dilation.

Cervical effacement is the thinning or shortening of the cervical walls (see diagram). It is measured by the percent to which the cervix has thinned: 0% defines a totally intact cervix and 100% means the cervix is paper thin. When the term "fully dilated" is used, it is also assumed that 100% cervical effacement has been achieved.

Sometimes you will hear the cervix described as "soft," which means it is in the process of dilation and effacement.

A PRIMIPARA is a woman who has never given birth before. The cervix of a primipara needs to be completely effaced in order for the opening to actively dilate.

A woman who has given birth previously is called a MULTIPARA. Her cervix will efface and dilate simultaneously. For this reason ensuing labors are often shorter.

In the GRAND MULTIPARA, a woman who has given birth five or more times, uterine pressure toward the end of pregnancy may cause a physiological opening with only minimal effacement and without contractions. Cervical dilation in this case does not indicate imminent delivery. Since this opening is caused by pressure and not contractions, it does not render a woman a *niddah*.[2]

CERVICAL EFFACEMENT AND DILATION

PRIMIPARA   MULTIPARA

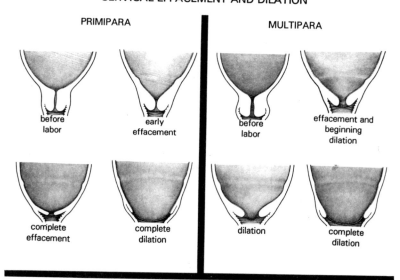

before   early   before   effacement and
labor   effacement   labor   beginning
                                                    dilation

complete   complete   dilation   complete
effacement   dilation   dilation

Another important measurement of progress in labor is the relation of the baby's head to a point in the woman's pelvis called the ISCHIAL SPINES. These are bony protuberances on both inner sides of the pelvis. The point parallel to the spines is designated "0." When the fetal head is above the spines it is labeled sp-1, -2, -3. When the baby has not yet entered the pelvic inlet (i.e., above sp-3), it is described as "floating." As labor progresses, the baby's head descends through sp-levels +1, +2, +3 and then passes through the pelvic outlet.

ISCHIAL SPINES
(Degree of Engagement)

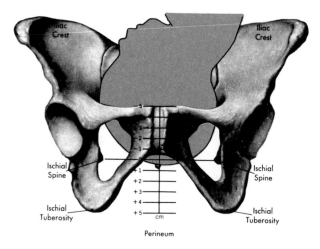

Reprinted with permission of Ross Laboratories, Columbus, Ohio
from "Clinical Education Aids"

ENGAGEMENT occurs when the baby's head has descended to the level of the ischial spines and fits snugly in the pelvis. Taut abdominal muscles will direct the baby's head into the pelvis before birth or shortly after the onset of labor. In primiparas, engagement can occur up to two weeks before delivery. This phenomenon is commonly termed "lightening" because the lower the baby is, the easier it is for the woman to breathe, eat, etc. However, it also causes increased pressure on the bladder which results in more frequent urination.

By the time labor starts in a primipara, the baby's head should already be engaged. If this is not the case, it could be an indication of possible disproportion between the baby's head and the mother's pelvis (large head vs. small pelvis), otherwise called cephalopelvic disproportion (CPD). In most cases, CPD requires cesarean section.

A multipara, whose abdominal muscles have been weakened, may start labor when the fetal head is still above the ischial spines or even above the pelvic inlet. The fetal head will, therefore, descend during labor. Sometimes in grand multiparas the head will only descend after full dilation, immediately preceding delivery.

With a fuller understanding of the three basic parameters for measuring the progress of delivery — dilation, effacement, and the descent of the fetal head — you will now be better able to understand descriptions of your progress in labor. This wil facilitate better communication and mutual cooperation between you and your caregivers.

Rupture of membranes (breaking of waters) and uterine contractions both signal the start of labor. If one or both of these symptoms appear, you should call your doctor or go directly to the hospital.

When to Go to the Hospital

RUPTURE OF MEMBRANES occurs when the membranes of the amniotic sac tear, releasing some of the amniotic fluid. The breaking of waters may or may not be accompanied by uterine contractions, even at term. When membranes rupture without contractions, there may as yet be no cervical dilation, and therefore the woman is not rendered a *niddah*. However, some *poskim* suspect that the discharge of amniotic fluid may have been accompanied by blood, and consider her a *niddah*. The husband should, therefore, refrain from physical contact with his wife unless she is in need of assistance.[3] It is not advisable to perform a *bedikah* to verify bleeding at this time because of the risk of infection.

If you are not sure whether your water has actually broken, here is a simple way to check: dry the perineal area and place a pad in your underwear, then check the pad after half an hour. If it is quite wet, this is a positive indication of ruptured membranes. You should seek medical attention within the hour.

UTERINE CONTRACTIONS require going to the hospital if they continue at 5-10 minute intervals for a minimum of one hour. These contractions usually make staying in one position uncomfortable. From this point you should consider yourself a *niddah*.[4] However, if you are in need of assistance, your husband may come to your aid.[5] (For further details, see following section listing characteristics of true labor.)

The decision to go to the hospital depends on previous labor experiences and how long it takes to get to the hospital. Many women feel more comfortable staying at home when they are in labor; others enjoy the reassuring atmosphere of a medical setting. Whichever you prefer, you can avoid unnecessary tension by not waiting too long before going to the hospital.

When considering the appropriate time to go to the hospital, women can be evaluated according to three specific categories:

First Birth: When contractions are every 3-5 minutes, last 30-60 seconds, and continue for at least one hour, the woman should go to the hospital.

Multipara: When contractions occur every 5 minutes, last 30-60 seconds, and continue at regular intervals for at least half an hour to an hour, the woman should go to the hospital.

Complications: Women who have had previous cesarean sections, unusual bleeding, high blood pressure, or abnormally severe pain are considered high-risk deliv-

eries. In addition, women who have a history of rapid deliveries or who live far from the hospital fall into this
category. Women in this category should go to the hospital after an hour of contractions which are 10 minutes
apart.

As mentioned in Chapter 10, not all uterine con-   **True vs.**
tractions signify the start of labor. Braxton Hicks   **False Labor**
(false) contractions are analogous to the uterus
flexing its muscles for the big event! False contractions
do not cause the cervix to dilate. They are often experienced
toward the end of pregnancy and occur more often when
the pregnant woman overworks or does not drink enough.

It is helpful to be able to differentiate between true
and false labor in order to avoid guesswork and a need-
less trip to the hospital.

False Labor	**True Labor**
‣ contractions felt in abdomen only	‣ contractions felt in back, sweeping forward toward the abdomen
‣ irregular intervals	‣ regular intervals
‣ mild	‣ increasingly stronger and painful
‣ no bloody show (see below)	‣ bloody show
‣ contractions fade with position-change or activity	‣ contractions continue no matter what the position or activity

[Bloody show is a slightly blood-tinged mucous discharge. It indicates that the mucous plug which has sealed the uterus throughout
pregnancy is breaking down due to the softening and effacement of the
cervix preceding labor. Although it is a sign of impending labor, it does
not require immediate medical attention.]

Some women experience a pre-labor phase, which   **Pre-Labor**
is a preparatory period that can precede true labor   **Phase**
and may last for days. It can become very annoy-
ing, especially as contractions may really hurt, yet stop
as suddenly as they start. There will be an increase in
vaginal discharge, but not a bloody show. You feel as

though something is about to happen — and it is! These pre-labor pangs signify that true labor is not far away.

Labor   Labor is technically divided into four stages:
1. from onset of labor until full dilation (10 cm.)
2. from full dilation until birth of baby
3. from birth of baby until delivery of the placenta
4. from delivery of placenta until one hour after birth

First Stage   The first stage of labor can be further divided into
of Labor   two phases: latent phase and active phase.

During the LATENT PHASE, there is minimal cervical dilation — from 0-4 cm. with effacement of up to 60-80%. Contractions are fairly regular and mild. They come at approximately 15- to 20-minute intervals and last for only about 45 seconds. The latent phase can continue for up to 20 hours in a primipara and 14 hours in a multipara.

When discussing labor, you may hear someone say she was in labor for two days, or 24 hours, and so on. That is not really accurate. Although the latent phase is true labor, it is not hard labor, and you are still quite able to move about or even sleep. Most women prefer to stay at home until contractions intensify.

In the ACTIVE PHASE, contractions are more regular, more intense, and more frequent, causing rapid cervical dilation and effacement. The active phase is in turn subdivided into two intervals: regular active and transition.

During the REGULAR ACTIVE segment, dilation progresses from 3 cm. to 8 cm., and 90-100% effacement is achieved. Contractions gradually build in strength and lengthen in duration (60-90 seconds), while becoming more frequent (5-10 minutes apart). The regular active interval, including transition, can last up to 8 hours in a primipara and 4 hours in a multipara.

TRANSITION is the bridge between the active segment of labor and full dilation. It is the shortest and most intense part of the active phase. Contractions intensify, coming in one- to three-minute intervals and lasting 60-90 seconds. The cervix completes its dilation to 10 cm.

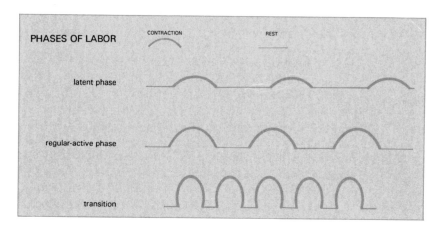

YOU AND THE HOSPITAL

The majority of women in labor come to the hospital while in the active phase. When you arrive at the hospital, your husband or escort will remain in the waiting area for a short time while you undergo the preliminary interview and examination.

The nurse or midwife will review your medical documents and ask pertinent questions. You will be examined internally to ascertain which stage of labor you have reached. The baby's heartbeat will also be checked.

If you are still in the latent phase of labor, the caregiver may suggest that you walk around for an hour or so and then return to be re-examined to determine if labor is progressing. You might have come to the hospital on a "false alarm." That's okay — it can happen to anybody. In such a case, a recording of the fetal monitor will be taken, and you will be sent home.

FALSE ALARM AND NIDDAH

If you are sent home from the hospital, and you have no cervical dilation, you are not considered a *niddah*. On the other hand, if your cervix has begun to dilate, even if you are sent home from the hospital, you are still considered *niddah*.[6]

ADMISSION TO THE HOSPITAL

If labor has progressed into the active phase, you will be admitted to the labor and delivery ward in accordance with each hospital's standard admission policy. Of course, if you are very close to giving birth, you will go straight to the birthing area, bypassing the admitting routine.

Admitting procedures do vary between hospitals, but certain standard practices can be expected. Some women will choose one hospital over another on the basis of the admission routine practiced at each hospital. Four of the most standard medical intervention practices are: shave, enema, intravenous, and fetal monitoring.

The SHAVE consists of removing the pubic hair around the perineal orifice to allow better visualization of the perineum. Seeing the area clearly helps the caregiver to prevent tearing and facilitates the performance of an episiotomy. (A cesarean section requires shaving the entire pubic area up to the umbilicus.)

It has not been proven that shaving is necessary or that it really promotes a more germ-free environment for healing (in normal deliveries), or even that it helps prevent infection. Therefore, a routine shave is often not performed. Many physicians, however, prefer a shaved perineum while performing episiotomies and suturing.

Many women welcome the shave for aesthetic reasons during the birth. It also makes it easier to cope with postpartum blood flow and discharges. Most hospitals are quite willing to forgo the shave for multiparas, as the chance of an episiotomy or of tearing is minimal. It is also perfectly acceptable for you to request that you not be shaved on Shabbos. The shave may always be done at a later stage, as deemed necessary by the midwife or doctor during the delivery.

The purpose of the ENEMA is to flush the lower segment of the large intestine of all fecal material. Warm soapy water (250 cc. to one liter) is introduced into the rectum by means of a narrow plastic tube. It is not painful, only mildly uncomfortable for approximately two minutes as the water fills the bowel. After the enema, you will need to walk around a little bit and then use the facilities at least 2-3 times before the bowel is completely empty.

At the same time that the smooth muscle of the intestine is stimulated by the enema, the smooth muscle of the uterus responds as well, and contractions may intensify. This may help labor to progress faster. Another advantage of the enema is the welcome relief it provides to the woman with constipation, a common annoyance at the end of pregnancy. Some women feel better knowing that the enema has forestalled the potential discomfort or embarrassment of passing stool while pushing during delivery. It is comforting to realize that, should it occur, professional caregivers would not be fazed at all, as it is quite commonplace.

It is perfectly acceptable to deliver without having an enema, and you should discuss any reservations you may have with your caregiver.

Many women wonder why they require INTRAVENOUS The most common reason to set up an intravenous line is to provide the fluids and glucose needed during labor. Since it is customary for a woman in labor not to eat or drink, an I.V. will replace the fluids and energy her body needs. However, you may forgo intravenous if the following conditions apply: you are not bedridden during labor; you want to walk around and can still do so; you are receiving no medication; and hospital policy permits.

At the same time the I.V. is inserted, blood will be withdrawn for routine blood tests during the course of labor. The I.V. can also be used to administer analgesic medication.

Although giving birth is not an illness, there is always a possibility of minor or even serious complications. Many hospitals and physicians regard an intravenous as an insurance policy to handle emergencies such as shock, high blood pressure and infection. In such cases, access to a vein will expedite treatment. It is the policy at some hospitals to insert an I.V. for a woman delivering her fifth child or more, as the chance of complications tends to rise from the fifth birth and upward.

As was discussed in the prenatal section of the book, FETAL MONITORING is beneficial in evaluating the baby's healthy response to uterine contractions. Most hospitals require at least one 20-minute baseline monitor at the start of labor. During labor, the baby may be monitored for a few minutes each hour, manually at frequent intervals, or continuously throughout labor. Your caregiver will decide how often to monitor, taking into consideration hospital policy and the condition of mother and baby.

Open communication between you and the hospital staff (and vice versa) is extremely important. When the hospital staff communicates and explains procedures, you feel informed, encouraged, reassured and secure. When you discuss your needs, concerns and desires with the hospital staff, you can actively participate in decision-making and improve the quality of the care you receive.

Some hospitals encourage the use of a pre-written care plan, while others may have steadfast rules. In general, however, if you present your wishes in a sincere and respectful manner, most nurses, midwives and doctors will welcome discussion and will work with you to make your labor and delivery experience a positive one.

After admission, you will be assigned to a labor room, which in most cases doubles as a delivery room. You do not necessarily have to get right into bed. Labor is a dynamic process in which conditions are constantly changing. You may continue to sit up or walk around as long as the following conditions apply: you are feeling strong, the fetal monitor is normal, the baby's head is engaged, and there are no medical problems. If you are in an upright position, you won't feel like a sick patient confined to bed, and you will also assist the labor process by taking advantage of the natural forces of gravity. In addition, moving about will keep muscles relaxed and blood circulating, and can also help distract you during contractions.

If you begin to feel extremely tired, or the pain seems to be overwhelming, this could be your body's signal to you to take it easy and lie down. Other circumstances in which you will be asked to remain in bed include: ruptured membranes without engagement of the baby's head, fetal distress, anesthesia, and maternal illness.

Once in bed, the position of choice is on your left side with your head slightly (30°) elevated. It is all right to lie on your right side as well, but it is definitely not recommended to lie flat on your back, as this position reduces the blood and oxygen supply to your body.

AMNIOTOMY

If the amniotic membranes have not ruptured spontaneously (your waters have not broken) before the active phase of labor, your caregiver may perform an amniotomy. The artificial rupture of the membranes (AROM) allows the amniotic fluid in front of the fetal head (forewaters) to be released, and then the baby's head should automatically descend to fit snugly against the cervix. Breaking the water is also necessary to facilitate internal monitoring of the fetal heartbeat or contractions. Uterine contractions usually strengthen after an amniotomy, and in some cases the first stage of labor may even be shortened.

After the membranes are ruptured, the fluid will be examined. Its color will indicate whether or not meconium is present in the amniotic fluid, which is a warning sign of potential fetal distress. (See fetal distress, pp. 162 164.)

HUSBAND DURING LABOR

Concerning your husband's presence in the delivery room during labor, there are certain *halachos* that you must be aware of. Your husband is forbidden to look at the area where the birth is actually taking place, and once you are considered *niddah*,[7] he is also forbidden to look at the parts of your body that are normally covered.[8] He should sit at the head of the bed during the birth, facing away from the proscribed area.

Most *poskim* agree that the husband is allowed to be in the room during labor, although some say he should wait outside during the delivery.[9] Some *poskim* suggest that although the *halachah* may permit the husband to be in the delivery room, it still may be considered immodest and is not the preferred custom. According to Rabbi Moshe Feinstein, the husband is allowed to stay in the room even during the delivery.[10]

Some authorities maintain that if the husband wants to stay in the delivery room merely to "experience" the delivery and is not there for the specific purpose of helping and comforting his wife, it is forbidden. But if his wife requests that he stay to encourage and comfort her, not only is it permitted, but he is obligated to do so.[11]

Although a woman in labor is considered a *niddah*, her husband may come to her aid during labor if there is no one else to assist her at that time.[12]

ALMOST READY

During transition, with the approach of full dilation, some women become nauseous and vomit. If this occurs, it is best to rinse out the mouth rather than to drink.

Another common manifestation which precedes the second stage is a premature urge to push. At this point the cervix is dilated to approximately 9 3/4 cm., with only small cervical borders remaining undilated. Even though you are so close to full dilation, it is still too soon to push. Pushing at this time would only cause swelling of the cervical borders and thus slow the progress of labor. It can even cause cervical tearing.

Not everyone experiences this premature urge to push. If it does occur, it is most common in first or second deliveries. In some cases during an internal exami-

My frame
was not hidden
from Thee,
when I was made
in secret...

TEHILLIM 139:15

FIFTH WEEK

length, 3/8 in. (1 cm.)

SIXTH WEEK

the central nervous
system is forming

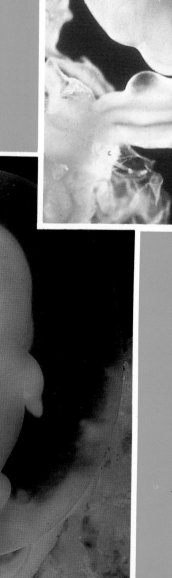

*His two eyes are
like the eyes of a fly
...His arms are like
strings of radiance.
His mouth like the
split of a barley, his
body like a lentil,
and his limbs are
connected like a
shapeless form. As
it is written, "Your
eyes have seen my
form."*

YERUSHALMI, NIDDAH 3:3

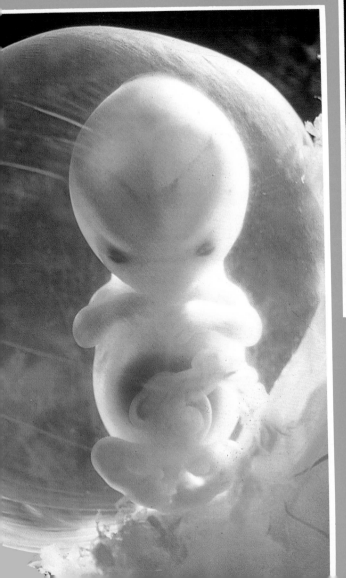

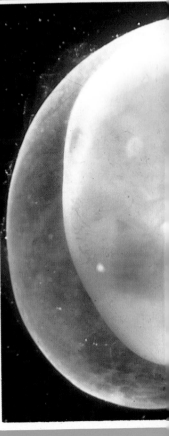

...Thou hast
knit me together
in my mother's
womb.

TEHILLIM 139:13

SEVENTH WEEK

length 3/4 in. (2 cm.)

*"From three to forty
days one should pray
for the specific gender
of the child..."*

I will praise Thee
for in an awesome,
wonderous way
did I come to be.

TEHILLIM 139:14

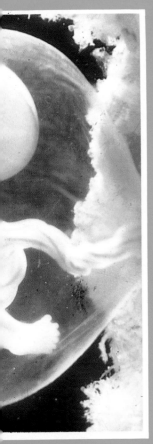

ELEVEN WEEKS

*"From forty days to three
months one should pray
that the baby not suffer
from any deformity..."*

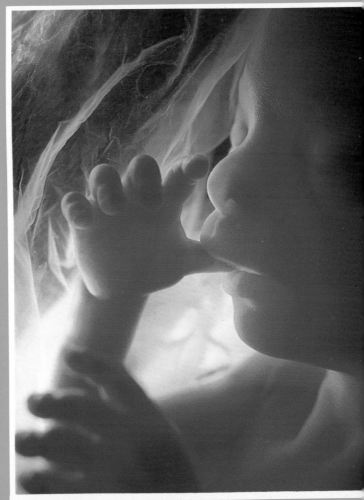

4-1/2 MONTHS

*"From three to six
months it is proper to
offer prayers that one
should not miscarry..."*

Photographs: Lennart Nilsson, *A Child Is Born*, ed. 1976

Marvelous are Thy works...
and my soul knows well.

TEHILLIM 139:14

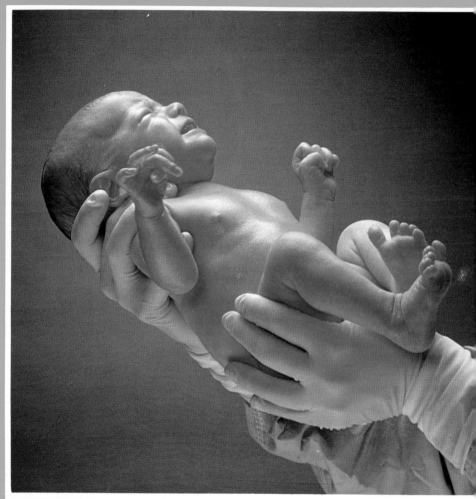

*"From six to nine months
one should pray that the
baby be delivered safely."*

BERACHOS 60a

nation, the midwife or doctor can literally lift the borders of the cervix (if they are thin and flexible) over the baby's descending head, enabling the second stage of labor to proceed.

Your caregiver will direct you by telling you when to push and when to refrain from pushing. If you are instructed not to push during a contraction, "pant-breathing" (breathing like a puppy) will help control this involuntary urge. To pant-breathe, inhale deeply and exhale in the following pattern:

HEH. . . HEH. . . HEH. . . WHOO

and repeat it for the duration of the contraction.

Second Stage of Labor

Following the transition segment of the active phase, the second stage of labor is often a welcome relief. The second stage can last anywhere from a few minutes to 1-2 hours. During this period, incessant waves of contractions give way to the urge to push, and, because the cervix is fully dilated, you can finally give in to that urge. In this way, you are able to constructively work along with the contractions and actually help your baby complete his journey into this world. Also, because your energy and concentration are so intently directed toward pushing, contractions are no longer painful.

The urge to push is caused by the pressure of the baby's head on the nerve endings in the pelvis. Despite your natural and reflexive desire to bear down at this time, you must control and coordinate your efforts with directives given by your caregiver. Uncontrolled pushing can propel the baby too rapidly through the birth canal, increasing the risk of head trauma for the baby and of perineal lacerations in the mother.

Controlled pushing can prevent trauma to both mother and baby. It also conserves your energy by allowing both pushing and resting when appropriate. Working together with your caregiver to push, or at times refrain from pushing, will also reduce the possible need for medical intervention.

HOW TO PUSH

Pushing properly is more efficient and can shorten the second stage of labor by half! This should be the primary message of any childbirth class. The following information is, nevertheless, provided as a reference guide to assist the woman in labor.

You may assume several different positions during the second stage of labor. One of these positions is left-side lying. As was previously mentioned, left-side lying facilitates the maximum blood and oxygen supply to the fetus. It also helps to direct the baby's head to the proper angle in the pelvis. As shown in the illustration, from the point the baby engages himself in the pelvic inlet to the point he exits the pelvic outlet, he is continuously rotating his head, making adjustments which expedite his descent through the birth canal. Since the circumference of the baby's head is the largest part of his body, he must maneuver himself in order to successfully

MECHANISM OF NORMAL LABOR

1.
Engagement,
Descent,
Flexion

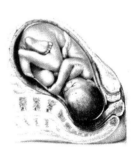

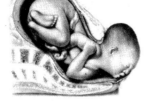

4.

Extension Complete

5.

External Rotation

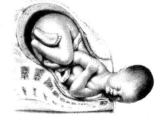

pass through the mother's pelvis. In addition to helping the progress of the baby's descent, left-side lying is safe and comfortable. For these reasons, women in England routinely deliver in this position.

You may feel you can push more effectively when squatting or sitting in a birthing chair. Squatting requires considerable physical stamina and adequate physical support. Using a birthing chair is similar to squatting. It positions you to push naturally, making use of the force of gravity, yet without the additional burden of having to support your own weight.

Lying flat on your back with your feet up in stirrups is not considered a good option. However, lying in bed with the torso raised to a 45° angle can be very comfortable. This semi-reclining position is used regularly in most hospitals. If a woman is calm and controlled and there are no medical complications, stirrups are not necessary.

2.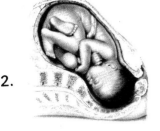

Internal Rotation

3.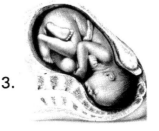

Extension Beginning

6.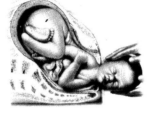

Shoulder Rotation

7.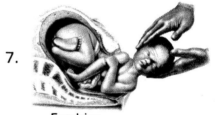

Expulsion

There are four steps to proper and effective pushing:

1. Take a long, deep breath at the start of the contraction.
2. Close your mouth and keep it closed while pushing. If you talk or make noises from your throat, your pushing will not be as effective as it can be.
3. Put your chin to your chest.
4. Bear down as if you are having a bowel movement.

You should be able to push about four times during each contraction. Each pushing effort can last as long as 10 seconds with a deep breath between each push.

It may be preferable to avoid pushing in one strong, continuous effort. Instead, a series of short, gentle pushes is more effective, especially when the baby's head has reached the vaginal opening (CROWNING). The short pushes ease the head out gradually, and thus an episiotomy or lacerations may be prevented. To push intermittently, simply open your mouth to breathe between short efforts. Again, your caregiver will give you specific directions about how and when to push.

Do not be afraid to change positions during the second stage in order to find the position which is most comfortable for you. Many women will lie on their left side and push until the baby's head crowns, and then turn to a semi-sitting position to deliver.

An EPISIOTOMY is an incision made in order to widen the vaginal opening. There are two types of episiotomies: the median, or midline episiotomy, which is a straight cut from the bottom of the vagina toward the rectum, and the medial-lateral episiotomy, which is cut on a diagonal. Each incision incorporates not only the surface tissue, but a layer of muscle. Therefore, after all deliveries, and even more so following the performance of an episiotomy, it is extremely important to exercise the muscles of the pelvic floor.

One advantage to performing an episiotomy is that the incision is straight and clean, whereas perineal tearing can be ragged and uncontrolled. An episiotomy also minimizes pressure on the baby's head as it crowns before birth. This is of special significance in cases of fetal distress, when a vacuum or forceps delivery is indicated, or when the baby weighs less than 5 lbs. (2.2 kg.) and is more susceptible to head trauma. Also, during a twins or breech delivery (see Chapter 14), an episiotomy allows the doctor greater maneuverability.

The episiotomy is made as the baby's head is crowning and the woman is pushing. Local anesthesia (lidocaine) may or may not be used. The mother usually does not feel the incision as the pressure of the fetal head against the perineum is so intense that the nerve endings are momentarily deadened.

An episiotomy is considered a normal part of a first delivery. For subsequent births, it is done less routinely because the perineum becomes more flexible and elastic. A primipara can also deliver without an episiotomy, provided she can maintain calm and controlled pushing, and is guided by a skilled midwife or doctor. Naturally, most women prefer not to have an episiotomy if possible, for this — as with any surgical incision — entails stitches and added discomfort during the brief healing process. Women who never develop a more elastic perineum, or have a build-up of scar tissue from a previous episiotomy, will need an episiotomy to avoid perineal tearing at every delivery.

THE BIRTH

In most cases the baby's head will emerge face down. When the whole head is out, the baby will spontaneously rotate to the side, allowing his shoulders to emerge one at a time. When the rest of the baby's body slips out, you will feel a great release of pressure.

Your newborn will be placed either on your stomach or on a small cart at the side of the bed. The baby's head and body will then be wiped clean of excess amniotic fluid, vernix and maternal blood to prevent rapid heat loss. The umbilical cord will be clamped and cut as the baby takes his first breaths of life. He should cry almost immediately — on his own or in response to gentle rubbing.

At this time your baby's respiratory and circulatory systems are making a monumental transformation from intrauterine life to life in our world. The blood of the fetus was shunted between the top chambers of the heart (right and left atrium) through a hole called the foramen ovale. The newborn needs to fully oxygenate his lungs, so the foramen ovale closes to allow the blood to circulate properly. The Gemara (*Niddah* 30b) clearly describes this process: "When the fetus sees the light [i.e., is born], the closed organ opens and the open one closes. For if this would not happen, the baby could not live even a single hour."

A TIME TO REFLECT

Shelomo *Ha-Melech* wrote in *Koheles*, "To everything there is a time; a time to every purpose under heaven: a time to be born. . ."

Everything has a proper time, and every new moment is significant. Yet, as mentioned in the beginning of this chapter, "the time to be born" — the start of life — seems to be the most special of all.

When we think of mankind reproducing and new generations replacing older ones, we may view it as a mundane fact of life. But on a personal level, when a child is born we are overcome with amazement at this astonishing "miracle that God has done for me." Each birth is indeed a miraculous occurrence that stirs our emotions and heightens our admiration and appreciation of *Hashem Yisbarach.*

On the verse, "He does countless wonders" (*Iyov* 9:9) the Midrash explains that this refers to the moment of birth. How fortunate is the woman who has merited a share in this great event. How fortunate is the mother who brings another Jewish soul into the world.

"Happy is the mother of her children" (*Tehillim* 113:9).

Though the baby has been born, it is customary to **Third Stage** delay saying *mazal tov* until the placenta has also **of Labor** been delivered. The placenta may not be expelled for as long as an hour after the birth.

Your caregiver may externally massage the uterus to facilitate delivery of the placenta. As it separates itself from the uterine wall, you may feel your uterus contract and a slight urge to push; however, you will not feel discomfort as the placenta slides through the birth canal. The placenta will be thoroughly checked to verify that no fragments have remained in the uterus, for this can cause hemorrhage and infection. If so, the fragments are removed manually.

At this stage the uterus will begin a series of therapeutic contractions aimed at preventing blood loss. You may once again receive an external massage to stimulate these contractions. Oxytocin may also be administered either intravenously or intramuscularly to further promote uterine contractions.

If stitches are required to repair an episiotomy or perineal tearing, suturing will be done at this time. If not, you will be rinsed and your bedding will be changed to make you more comfortable.

It is customary to wash your hands (*netilas yadayim*) at this point, especially if you want to eat and drink. The reason for washing is that it is likely that during the course of labor you touched parts of your body which are normally covered.[13]

Many Ashkenazim customarily recite a *berachah* of gratitude for the birth of a child. The *berachah* of *ha-tov v'ha-metiv* is said for the birth of a boy, and for the birth of a girl, *shehecheyanu*.[14] The mother and father should each say the *berachah*.[15] The *berachah* should be said as soon as possible after the delivery room has been cleaned. The father should recite the *berachah* as soon as he hears of the birth, even if he has not yet seen the baby. But if the *berachah* was not said immediately, it may still be said as long as the birth still feels new.[16]

According to Sephardic custom, no *berachah* is recited until the *bris milah*, when the father says *shehecheyanu*. At that time, he should have in mind the
birth of his son.[17]

During the third stage, the observation and care of
your newborn will continue. His nostrils and mouth may
be suctioned gently to remove excess amniotic fluid in-
haled at the birth.

One minute after birth and again at five minutes,
your baby will be evaluated according to the Apgar rating system, and given a score. The Apgar score is a uni-
form rating system for evaluating the well-being of a
baby at birth. The baby's heart rate, respiration, muscle
tone, reflexes, and color are checked and rated on a
scale of 0 to 2. These numbers are then added up to give
the total Apgar score (10 being the best possible score).

Apgar Score

CRITERIA	0	1	2
COLOR	blue, pale	body pink, extremities blue	all pink
HEART RATE	absent	less than 100	more than 100
RESPIRATION	absent	irregular, slow	good, crying
REFLEX (to suctioning)	none	grimace	sneeze, cough
MUSCLE TONE	limp	some flexion of extremities	active

Additional care of the newborn will be carried out in
the delivery room on a heated bassinet or later in the
newborn nursery. Your baby's weight and length will be
measured and documented, and two or three identifica-
tion bracelets will be placed on his ankles and wrists.

Initial medical treatment of the newborn includes administering silver nitrate drops or antibiotic ointment to
his eyes to prevent gonorrheal conjunctivitis. Although
this practice is virtually obsolete, it is usually mandated
by law. Recently, many areas of the world have dropped
this procedure, and you may inquire what the policy is

at your local hospital. Another treatment for the newborn is Vitamin K, administered intramuscularly to assist the function of the immature coagulation system.
(For a more detailed look at newborn care, refer to Chapter 19 on The Newborn.)

The first hour after delivery is a critical time for **Fourth Stage**
both mother and baby. Your newborn's respiration **of Labor**
and temperature will be carefully observed, while
your blood pressure will be monitored. The uterus will be
palpated at designated intervals to verify that it is contracting and that blood loss is minimal.

During this hour, you may nurse the baby for the
first time, if you so desire. Breast feeding will cause a
natural release of the hormone oxytocin, which speeds
the contraction of the uterus. Immediately following a
delivery, it is also standard procedure to administer oxytocin in its synthetic form, pitocin, either intramuscularly or through an I.V.

An hour after the birth you will be encouraged to urinate. It may take longer for you to control urination if
you have had an epidural. In addition to not feeling the
urge to urinate, having to use a bedpan can be inhibiting. It is a good idea to request assistance to sit up in
bed over the bedpan. This more natural position can facilitate urination. Also, rinsing the perineum with water
can promote the urge to urinate.

Some women experience trembling and chills. This is
a common occurrence and can be quickly alleviated with
an extra blanket and a warm drink. If you are hungry,
feel free to eat and drink as you wish.

This relaxed time after birth is often the most beautiful and emotional part of the entire experience. Mother,
father, and newborn are united as a family for the first
time. You and your husband will want to share your
thoughts and feelings, maybe have a good laugh or cry.
God willing, this is the start of many years of joy and
happiness for all.

NOTES

1. *Ta'anis* 2a.
2. According to R. Mordechai Eliyahu and R. Chaim P. Sheinberg; *see* Chazon Ish, *Yoreh De'ah* 83:1.
3. *See* Hebrew appendix.
4. *Sidrei Taharah* 194:25; *see Iggros Moshe, Yoreh De'ah*, vol. II, 75.
5. Rama, *Yoreh De'ah* 195:16.
6. According to *Sidrei Taharah* 194:25; *see* Hebrew appendix. In a case where the false contractions caused an opening a few weeks before the due date, a Rav should be consulted.
7. Real contractions render a woman *niddah.*
8. *Yoreh De'ah* 195:7; *Orach Chayim* 240:4.
9. *Minchas Yitzchak*, vol. VIII, 30; however, he allowed it in the event of great necessity; *see also* R. Mordechai Eliyahu, *Darkei Taharah*, p. 111.
10. *Iggros Moshe, Yoreh De'ah*, vol. II, 75; *see also* R. Ovadyah Yosef, *Taharas Ha-Bayis*, vol. II, p. 166, who also says that it is permissible.
11. R. *Yehudah Herzl Henkin, Assia*, vol. II, p. 117.
12. Rama, *Yoreh De'ah* 195:16; *see Toras Ha-Yoledes* 31, notes 3-5; *see also Badei Ha-Shulchan* 194, *biurim* p. 251.
13. *Orach Chayim* 4:19; *Mishnah Berurah* 46.
14. *Orach Chayim* 223:1; *Mishnah Berurah* 2 and 7; *Tzitz Eliezer*, vol. XIII, 20.
15. *Tzitz Eliezer*, vol. XIV, 22.
16. *Mishnah Berurah* 223:1-3; *Kaf Ha-Chayim* 227:5, 330. If the father was not present at the birth of his son, he should recite the *berachah* as soon as he hears of the birth. If he was not present at the birth of his daughter, *see* Hebrew appendix.
17. Ben Ish Chai, first year, *Parashas Re'eh*; *Kaf Ha-Chayim* 223:6.

14 | Special Considerations in Labor and Delivery

Even there shall Your hand lead me and Your right hand shall hold me.

TEHILLIM 139:10

In most cases labor and delivery proceed smoothly, without problems. Occasionally, however, complications will arise.

Occipital Posterior Presentation

In normal births the baby presents facing the back of the mother (i.e., the baby is born facing down). In about 5% of all deliveries, the fetal head maneuvers itself so that the occiput (back) faces the back of the mother (i.e., the baby is born with his face directed upwards). In such cases, labor can take a bit longer and is characterized by increased back pain and pressure.[1] An episiotomy is usually necessary, and there is a greater likelihood of forceps or vacuum delivery (see below).

Breech Presentations

During the early part of pregnancy, the majority of fetuses lie in a breech position (the baby is vertical with the legs or buttocks presenting towards the birth canal). By the 34th week of gestation, however, the fetus generally turns to present its head towards the birth canal. In about 3% of all deliveries, the fetus remains in the breech position.[2]

There are three types of breech presentation: Frank breech, complete breech, or footling breech (see illustration on page 159). A Frank breech may be delivered vaginally, while a footling breech and most complete breech presentations require delivery of the baby by cesarean section.

If the breech presentation persists until active labor, the situation is evaluated to ascertain if a cesarean section is necessary. Six factors are rated on a scale of 0-2, and this analysis is known as the Zatuchni Score (see chart). If the result is 0-3 points, a C-section is indicated. With a score of four points, the woman will be given a 2-hour trial of labor, to see if she can deliver normally. If her total is five or higher, she will be allowed to attempt to deliver normally unless a further difficulty arises.

Zatuchni Score

CRITERIA	0	1	2
PARITY	1st birth	multipara	
AGE OF PREGNANCY	39 weeks or more	38 weeks	37 weeks
PREVIOUS BREECH DELIVERY	none	1	2 or more
WEIGHT OF FETUS	7.702 lb. (3.501 kg.) or more	6.602-7.7 lb. (3.001-3.500 kg.)	5.502-6.6 lb. (2.501-3.000 kg.)
DILATION	2 cm.	3 cm.	4 cm.
LEVEL OF BREECH (ischial spines)	-3	-2	-1

In addition to a routine ultrasound, an x-ray is taken to determine the exact position of the breech. The x-ray will also determine the size of the baby's head and will reveal if it is flexed (bent forward) or extended back. In any presentation, the head needs to be flexed toward the chest in order to pass through the birth canal. The diameter of the baby's head is then compared to that of the mother's pelvis to rule out any disproportion which would inter-

CATEGORIES OF PRESENTATION

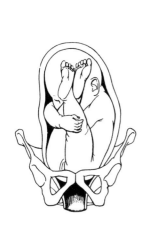

Frank Breech

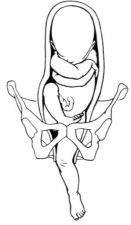

Footling Breech

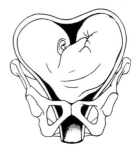

Shoulder Presentation

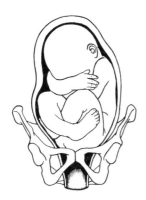

Complete Breech

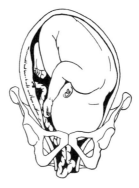

Prolapse of Cord

fere with delivery. In case of a previous cesarean section, a breech presentation would rule out vaginal delivery.

Vaginal delivery with a breech presentation takes more time than a normal delivery, as the baby's buttocks do not exert the same pressure on the cervix as the head does. Hospitals usually stipulate that two obstetricians preside over a breech delivery, and a pediatrician be on hand to examine the newborn immediately after birth.

Shoulder Presentation   Shoulder presentation (transverse lie) occurs only once in about 400 deliveries,[3] and usually in cases of prematurity, multiple birth, too much amniotic fluid (polyhydramnios), seriously reduced muscle tone of the mother's abdominal wall, or a contracted maternal pelvis. Once labor has begun and the baby continues to maintain the shoulder presentation, labor will not be allowed to proceed, and a cesarean section will be done.

External Version   External version is a technique practiced by some physicians in order to turn the baby to a position where it can be born head first. It is usually performed between week 32 and 36 of gestation. If successful, abdominal manipulation in a clockwise motion can rotate the baby's head into the pelvis, where it should remain until birth. However, there are instances when the fetus reverts to its original position.[4]

External version is not a simple procedure, and it may involve risks such as premature delivery or cord complications. It is contraindicated when the woman has previously delivered by cesarean section, her Rh factor is negative, or membranes have already ruptured.

Multiple Birth   Twins occur once in 83 pregnancies; triplets once in every 8,000 pregnancies; and quadruplets once in 400,000.[5] The occurrence of quintuplets, sextuplets and septuplets is rare and is usually the result of overstimulation of the ovaries through fertility drugs.

Identical twins (monozygotic) develop from one ovum

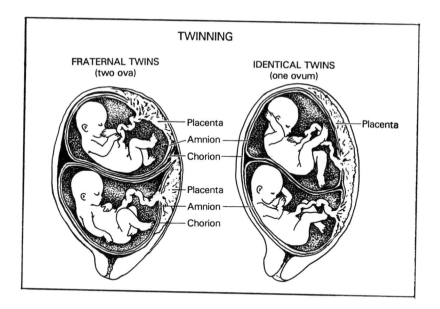

TWINNING

FRATERNAL TWINS
(two ova)

IDENTICAL TWINS
(one ovum)

Placenta
Amnion
Chorion

Placenta
Amnion
Chorion

Placenta

fertilized by one sperm, which then divides into two identical fertilized ova. They are, therefore, similar in physical and mental characteristics, and are always of the same sex. There is just one placenta between them.

Fraternal twins (dizygotic) are three times more common than identical twins. They are the result of two eggs released from the ovary at the same time, with each being fertilized by a different sperm. The babies may or may not be of the same sex, and their physical and mental characteristics can be as different as any two members of one family. Dizygotic twins are hereditary through the mother's family.

The word "more" is the key word in managing a multiple pregnancy. The expectant mother must make sure to enrich her diet, placing special emphasis on *more* protein, iron and folic acid. *More* fluids are also needed to help prevent premature contractions, which are so common in multiple pregnancies. And *more* rest is also necessary during such a pregnancy.

While the average pregnancy ends at about 39 weeks, twins are usually delivered at 35 weeks and triplets at 33 weeks. Pre-term delivery is, therefore, a major concern in multiple pregnancies.[6] In 50% of twin deliveries, both babies present head first.[7] The second baby should be born within 15 minutes of the birth of the first twin. If the second twin is situated in a transverse lie, external version is often attempted. In many instances the obstetrician will choose to employ internal version, reaching inside the uterus to turn the second twin to breech position to be delivered.

Multiple births are usually delivered in the operating room, with two obstetricians and an anesthesiologist present in case an emergency cesarean section is required. Two pediatricians are also on hand to care for the newborns.

Fetal Distress When the fetal heartbeat falls below or rises above the normal range (120-160), it is often a sign that the baby is in distress. Fetal distress is a catch-all term used whenever an abnormal heart rate indicates that the fetus might be suffering. It is often possible to resolve the problem by simply repositioning the mother on her left side or administering oxygen.

There are many possible causes of fetal distress:

HYPOXIA means the lack of oxygen. Hypoxia can be caused by compression of the umbilical cord, which reduces or even cuts off the flow of oxygen to the fetus. The umbilical cord may be entangled around the fetus or there may be a knot in the cord. In 2 to 3 babies out of 10, the umbilical cord is wrapped around the baby's neck. In most cases, these babies are delivered normally, without complications. Since the exact cause of hypoxia cannot always be determined during labor, the type of medical intervention needed depends upon the severity of the symptoms (e.g., changes in heart rate).

PROLAPSE of the umbilical cord is a condition where the cord presents before the baby's head, becoming compressed against the cervical opening. This fairly uncommon situation constitutes a medical emergency, and a cesarean section must be performed within minutes to prevent brain damage or worse. Prolapse of the cord can occur when the waters have broken and the fetal head is not engaged (fitted snugly in the pelvis). For this reason, many health professionals recommend bed rest once the waters have broken.

There can also be an "occult" (unseen) prolapse of the umbilical cord, when any part of the baby presses against the cord. This can resolve itself with a change in the mother's position, which often shifts the fetus away from the umbilical cord. If the condition is not resolved, medical intervention may be required.

SECOND STAGE DECELERATION: During the second stage of labor, slight decelerations in the fetal heart rate may occur while the mother pushes. As the baby's head comes through the cervix, his oxygen supply is reduced, and consequently his heart rate is lowered. This is considered a normal occurrence during the second stage. As long as the baby's heart rate returns to normal at the end of the contraction (conclusion of pushing), no medical intervention is required.

MATERNAL INFLUENCES, such as low blood pressure, hemorrhage, fever, or dehydration, can affect the fetal heart rate.

MECONIUM STAINING in the amniotic fluid is another warning sign of fetal distress. As mentioned previously, meconium is fecal material present in the fetal intestines, which normally is not excreted until after birth. The premature release of meconium into the amniotic fluid indicates that the fetus is suffering and requires diligent monitoring.

pH SAMPLING is sometimes used to determine the severity of fetal distress. A .5 cc. sample of fetal blood is taken from the baby's scalp after the waters have broken and the baby's head is accessible. The normal pH of blood is 7.35, and brain cells will die if the pH drops below 7.0. Termination of labor is considered if the pH reaches 7.2 or lower.

Forceps and Vacuum Delivery Sometimes extra medical assistance is required in the form of a forceps or vacuum delivery. This may be indicated for a woman who is having a prolonged and difficult second stage of labor, where the ability to push is impaired due to epidural anesthesia, exhaustion, hysteria, or inadequate pushing skills. It may also be required in cases of heart disease, high blood pressure or other illnesses, where pushing is contraindicated. And, when there are signs of fetal distress and rapid delivery is required, a forceps or vacuum delivery may be deemed necessary to hasten the birth.

An assisted delivery will be performed only when the cervix is fully dilated and the membranes are ruptured. There can also be no evidence of disproportion between the fetal head and the maternal pelvis (cephalopelvic disproportion — CPD). An episiotomy is usually required with a forceps or vacuum delivery.

Forceps are rounded stainless steel blades resembling kitchen tongs. The obstetrician grips the fetal head between the two blades and slowly rotates and pulls the baby's head through the outlet of the pelvis, past the perineum.

The vacuum extractor is a suction cup attached to a tube leading to a pressure regulator. The cup is attached to the baby's head. Then gentle traction is applied, while the obstetrician pulls the baby past the perineum.

Nowadays, forceps are used less often than in previous years. They have been replaced by the less traumatic vacuum extractor and by the rising rate of cesarean section.

Post-Date Ten percent of all pregnancies continue past the standard textbook due date of 40 weeks' gestation. From 41 weeks, the pregnancy is considered post-date. Being overdue can cause some women a great deal of anxiety, while others take the extra week or two in stride.

The major concern in post-date pregnancy is the diminishing quantity of amniotic fluid. The amount of amniotic fluid can drop considerably after the 40th week of pregnancy (from the 500-1500 ml. to 400 ml. at week 42).[8] This fluid reduction (oligohydramnios) decreases the natural cushioning effect needed to protect the baby during contractions.

Another danger in post-date pregnancy is placental aging. Toward the end of the pregnancy the placenta loses some of its ability to function. It develops fibrotic, fatty deposits, which prevent the fetus from receiving sufficient oxygen and nutrients, thus endangering its life.

The diagnosis of post-maturity must take many factors into consideration. Dates can be inaccurate; immersion in the *mikveh* may have occurred later than usual; and sometimes ovulation is delayed. All of these factors can alter a due date. Ultrasound examinations at intervals throughout the pregnancy validate the accuracy of the projected due date.

A woman does not need to go to the hospital immediately after her due date passes, as long as she regularly feels her baby moving. Three to four days after her due date, however, she should seek medical attention. She will then undergo fetal monitoring every two to three days to confirm the baby's well-being.

An ultrasound may also be done to measure the amount of amniotic fluid, to observe the baby's respiration and general movements, and to estimate birth weight. This is referred to as a biophysical profile. Based on the result of the biophysical profile, a woman may be allowed to continue the pregnancy until labor begins spontaneously, or until any compromise in the baby's health is detected. If there is any danger to the baby, labor will be induced.

The rate of cesarean section in post-date pregnancies is generally higher than the norm.

Induction of Labor — the Torah View

Inducing labor is permissible only if it is dangerous to the mother or fetus to continue the pregnancy. This halachic ruling was made by Rabbi Moshe Feinstein in his responsa, *Iggros Moshe*,[9] and also by Rabbi Ovadyah Yosef in *Taharas Ha-Bayis*.[10] It can also be understood in the overall perspective of Jewish philosophy, for Hashem keeps an exact calculation of when a person should come into and leave this world.

An example of this is the story of the birth of the twins, Ya'akov and Esav. Rivkah *Immenu* had a nine-month pregnancy, as opposed to Tamar, who carried her twins for only six months. The commentaries explain that Tamar was carrying two righteous people and wanted them to be born as soon as possible. Rivkah, on the other hand, was giving birth to one child who would be righteous and another who would be evil. She was, therefore, not as anxious for an early birth. We also learn later that Avraham *Avinu* died at the time Esav turned thirteen, before he became evil. Hashem wanted to spare Avraham the agony of seeing how wicked his grandson would become, and therefore brought Avraham to Heaven before his time. Thus Avraham's death was dependent on the timing of Esav's birth. The shorter Rivkah's pregnancy, the sooner Avraham would have died.[11]

Another reason can be deduced from the Talmud's statement that the baby's existence in the mother's womb is the best time of his life. It would, therefore, be unfortunate to shorten this very special time.[12]

Induction of Labor Labor may be induced because of a mother's ill health, premature rupture of membranes, or fetal distress. The two most common chemical agents used to induce labor are Prostaglandin E (gel or suppositories), and an intravenous drip of pitocin.

Prostaglandin is a neutral fatty acid generally present in the body chemistry. When it is introduced into the cervical area, it causes the cervix to soften and dilate more easily. Contractions may begin as a direct result of the application of prostaglandin or when pitocin is administered a few hours after the prostaglandin has been applied.

Pitocin is a synthetic form of the hormone oxytocin

which causes the uterus to contract. It is carefully administered using a special intravenous apparatus which delivers only a few drops per minute.

Induced labor generally causes the rapid onset of strong contractions. There is no gradual build-up as in normal labor. When labor is induced, therefore, most women need some form of pain relief. In a primipara especially, induction is usually a long process, and epidural anesthesia is recommended.

During an induction, the woman undergoes constant monitoring to observe the frequency and strength of contractions, as well as the baby's response to them.

Artificial rupture of membranes (amniotomy) is sometimes employed as a physical form of inducing labor. "Stripping," gently rubbing the cervical opening, is another physical means to stimulate labor. The rubbing widens the cervical opening and causes a partial disengagement of the amniotic membrane from the cervix. It does not actually break the waters, but it does cause a natural secretion of prostaglandin. Stripping may be done during a pelvic examination, and usually results in slight bleeding. This procedure renders the woman a *niddah*.[13]

When the administration of oxytocin, stripping or amniotomy is performed while labor is already in progress, it is referred to as "augmentation of labor." The purpose of augmentation is to increase the frequency or strength of the contractions. Augmentation is halachically permissible.

Cesarean Section

Cesarean section is an operation to remove the fetus through an incision in the abdominal wall and uterus. Millions of women and babies have been saved through the performance of cesarean section. This procedure is not a modern medical technique, but is an ancient surgical operation. Even the Mishnah discusses cesarean sections, in conjunction with halachic rulings concerning *tumas niddah*.[14]

Incisions: Low Transverse vs. Classical The abdominal wall can be cut in two ways: a vertical midline incision or a low horizontal incision above the pubic hair line (bikini incision). It is the type of cut to the uterine wall, however, which is of greatest significance for future pregnancies and deliveries. The two major types of uterine incisions are the Lower Segment Cesarean Section (LSCS) or the Classical Cesarean Section.

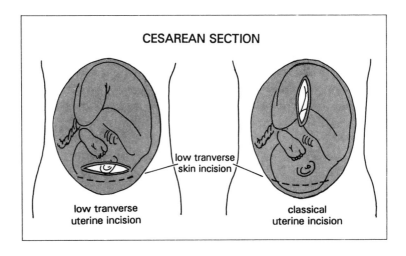

The lower segment cesarean section is the uterine incision of choice because less blood is lost than with a classical uterine incision. The LSCS is a horizontal incision in the lower part of the uterus. It allows a woman to deliver vaginally in subsequent births because future labor will not stress the healed suture line. The "Cohen cut," another version of the LSCS, is an incision very slightly higher, which is quicker to perform and repair.

The Classical incision is a vertical cut made from the lower uterine segment upward toward the fundus. Because of the threat of rupturing the previous classical cesarean scar during active labor, any subsequent delivery must be by cesarean section.

The following conditions often indicate a cesarean section:

fetal distress

failure of labor to progress (dystocia — the cervix
   does not dilate in response to uterine contractions)

previous C-section with classical incision

maternal infection (active herpes lesions)

unusual presentation (transverse, breech, or if the
   head presents by the face, brow or is flexed back)

large baby (after trial of labor)

cephalopelvic disproportion (CPD)

placenta previa (the placenta either partially or totally
   covers the cervical opening)

abruptio placentae (premature separation of the
   placenta from the uterine wall)

multiple births

prolapse of the umbilical cord

Failure to progress in labor accounts for the majority of all cesareans.[15]

Many factors influence the decision to perform a cesarean section. In addition to the clear-cut medical indications, an older primipara, an overly fearful woman, or a woman with a previous low-transverse cesarean section will also be considered for surgery. Every hospital and obstetrician has certain policies and opinions regarding the performance of cesarean sections. These should be investigated in advance by women who are potential candidates for a C-section.

Anesthesia in Cesarean Section

An EPIDURAL is the anesthesia of choice for cesarean section. It allows the woman to remain awake and aware throughout the entire procedure. She feels no pain, only slight pressure on her abdomen. Recovery is also easier, which gives her the chance to assume her "motherly" role more quickly.

GENERAL ANESTHESIA puts a woman to "sleep" for the entire operation. Nowadays it is usually reserved for emergency C-sections where saving time is an important consideration. Sometimes the anesthesiologist or the woman herself may have a preference for general anesthesia.

Preparation for Surgery Whether the cesarean section is elective (pre-planned) or an emergency decision, certain standard preparatory procedures are performed:

signed consent form
blood tests and cross-match for blood type in case a
    blood transfusion is needed
shaving of the stomach from the umbilicus to the pubic
    area
enema (only in an elective C-section)
intravenous line

Many women are allowed to come into the hospital the morning of an elective C-section. This provides a comfortable night at home before surgery. No food or drink should be consumed from midnight, the night before surgery.

Operating Room Some hospitals allow the husband to accompany his wife into the operating room for a cesarean. The operating room is kept at a low temperature to prevent germ proliferation. A woman should not hesitate to ask for a blanket if she feels chilly.

The woman's abdomen will be washed with an antiseptic solution, and the lower body will be draped with sterile linen. At this point, the epidural will have already been inserted or general anesthesia begun. After the anesthesia takes effect, a urinary catheter is inserted into the bladder. The medical team will monitor the fluid balance in relation to the urinary output. The woman will also be given oxygen through a mask to further oxygenate her baby.

The actual time from the start of the operation until the baby is born is 7-12 minutes. The remaining 50 minutes are spent suturing the uterus and abdomen.

Once the baby is born, a pediatrician will examine the newborn. If the new mother is awake and aware, she will be shown her new baby, thereby giving the bonding process a head start.

During the week after surgery, the healing and recovery process is remarkable. Every day is a milestone of improvement. The new mother gains strength and resumes responsibility for her own care as well as that of her baby.

Post-Operative Care and Recovery

The first 24 hours after surgery, a woman will be given pain relief through the epidural or, in the case of general anesthesia, by intramuscular injections. The urinary catheter will remain in place until she can walk to the bathroom on her own.

Getting out of bed within the first 12-24 hours will hasten recovery. Moving about is not only psychologically uplifting, but also helps the body systems return to normal. In addition, it facilitates the release of excess gas, which accumulates as a result of the general anesthesia "shutting down" the digestive tract for several hours.

As the intestines "wake up" after surgery, the new mother will be able to eat and drink again, and the intravenous will be removed. It is recommended to drink plenty of fluids, and eat fruit, vegetables, dried fruit and other foods which prevent constipation.

A post-cesarean mother can nurse comfortably by being propped up slightly with some pillows or cushions.

The incision is closed with stitches or clips (surgical staples), which will be removed 5-7 days after surgery. The incision site is very tender, and it is recommended to brace oneself with a pillow over the abdomen to prevent strain when laughing or coughing.

Postpartum bleeding is the same as for a woman after a vaginal delivery. This is a natural part of the uterine healing process after childbirth.

The average length of hospitalization is from 6-8 days.

If a woman had a cesarean birth on Shabbos, the *bris*

is not performed on the following Shabbos, as would be the case in a regular birth. The *bris* is postponed to the next day.[16]

If a firstborn son is delivered by cesarean section, no *pidyon ha-ben* is performed.[17]

The "Once a Cesarean. . ." Myth
Since 1978, there has been a growing trend to allow a woman who has previously given birth by cesarean section a trial of labor in her subsequent delivery. Vaginal birth after cesarean (VBAC) is an option that should be offered to all women who have undergone a low-transverse C-section and show no recurrent obstetrical reason for cesarean section.[18] The overall success rate for vaginal delivery after a cesarean is approximately 79%.[19] Even women who had a cesarean section due to failure to progress in labor are successful 61% of the time in delivering normally in subsequent pregnancies.[20]

Some progressive health care institutions even offer VBAC for women with two previous cesarean sections.

Any woman contemplating VBAC should choose a doctor who agrees with the possibility in principle. The hospital should also have a flexible VBAC policy and feature facilities for emergency services, an anesthesiologist on the premises, and blood bank services, should an emergency cesarean become necessary.

A cesarean birth should never be viewed as a disappointment. Hashem plans everything that occurs in our lives, and we should look at the ultimate good, that mother and child are alive and well. Whether or not the delivery was with or without medical intervention is immaterial. When we ask ourselves what the real goals of labor and delivery are, the answer should simply be: a healthy mother and baby.

NOTES

1. D.N. Danforth, *Obstetrics and Gynecology* (Philadelphia: Harper & Row, 1982), p. 700.
2. J.V. Collea, "Current Management of Breech Presentation," *Clinical Obstetrical Gynecology*, 23(2):525, 1980.
3. F.G. Cunningham, P.C. MacDonald, N.F. Gant, *Williams Obstetrics* (Norwalk: Appleton and Lange, 1989), p. 360.
4. B.M. Hibbard, *Principles of Obstetrics* (London: Butterworths, 1988), p. 562.
5. Mil, Pernoll, eds., *Current Obstetrics and Gynecology Diagnosis and Treatment* (Norwalk: Appleton and Lange, 1991), p. 352.
6. D.M. Campbell, I. MacGilliray, B. Thompson, eds., *Twinning and Twins* (Chichester: John Wiley & Sons Ltd., 1988), p. 143.
7. H. Oxorn, *Human Labor and Birth* (Norwalk: Appleton-Century-Crofts, 1986), p. 312.
8. F.C. Miller, J.A. Read, "Intrapartum Assessment of the Postdate Fetus," *American Journal of Obstetrics and Gynecology* 141:516, 1981.
9. *Iggros Moshe, Yoreh De'ah*, vol. II, 74.
10. *Taharas Ha-Bayis*, vol. II, p. 54.
11. See *Toras Ha-Yoledes*, ch. 1, note 1; and, in the name of Rabbi Y. S. Elyashiv, because it says in *Pirkei Avos* "for against your will you were created, against your will you were born...", the time of birth should be left up to the Creator of the universe.
12. *Niddah* 30b.
13. See *Pischei Teshuvah Yoreh De'ah* 134:4; *see also Iggros Moshe Orach Chayim*, vol. III, §100.
14. *Niddah* 40a.
15. E.J. Quilligan, F.P. Zuspan, *Douglas-Stromme Operative Obstetrics*, (Norwalk: Appleton and Lange, 1988), p. 476.
16. *Shulchan Aruch, Yoreh De'ah* 266:10; *see also Gemara Shabbos* 135a.
17. *Shulchan Aruch, Yoreh De'ah* 305:24.
18. B.L. Flamm, "Vaginal Birth after Cesarean Section: Controversies Old and New," *Clinical Obstetrics and Gynecology*, 28:735, 1985.
19. Ibid.
20. J. Seitchik and V. Rao, "Cesarean Delivery in Nulliparous Women for Failed Oxytocin-Augmented Labor," *American Journal OB/GYN*, 143:393, 1982.

15 | Shabbos in the Hospital

*Whoever brings delight to the Sabbath is
granted an inheritance without
constrictions.*
SHABBOS 118a

Many women may have to spend the Shabbos after delivery in the hospital. Rather than feeling depressed about
not being at home, take a look at the brighter side of
spending Shabbos in the hospital. As most hospitals
work with a skeleton crew on Shabbos, the staff has less
time for routine procedures such as taking temperatures
every four hours. You may, therefore, have the opportunity to catch up on some much-needed rest. Other advantages to being in the hospital over Shabbos are the
extra time you will have to spend with your baby, and
greater permissiveness with regard to visiting hours.

Before delivery, you should acquaint yourself with the
halachos that apply to every hospitalized patient on
Shabbos, to enable you to have the most enjoyable and
traditional Shabbos possible.

Lighting Although your husband may be lighting candles at
Candles home, you should nevertheless light candles in the
hospital.[1] It is preferable to light in the place where
you will eat.[2] In other words, if you eat in your room,
light candles there.

Outside Eretz Yisrael, lighting candles in the hospital can be problematic. When no candles are available, or if the hospital's fire laws prohibit lighting candles, some authorities have ruled that the woman can make a *berachah* on an electric light bulb (but not a fluorescent). Others say that she may turn on the light but not make a *berachah*.[3]

In Eretz Yisrael, most hospitals are far more flexible regarding candlelighting and women routinely light candles there.

When eating in the room: The law is different for Ashkenazi and Sephardi women. Sephardi women do not say a *berachah* on additional light, so if someone else lights before them in the same room, there is no longer any obligation for them to light. In other words, only one woman may light with a *berachah*.[4] Ashkenazi women, however, may light with a *berachah* even if other women have already lit in the same room.[5]

When there is one Sephardi woman and the others are Ashkenazi, it is preferable for the Sephardi woman to light first with a *berachah*. Afterwards, the Ashkenazi women may also light their Shabbos candles with a *berachah*.[6] If there is more than one Sephardi woman in the room, then only one of them should light with a *berachah*.

When eating in a dining hall: Ashkenazi women may light there with a *berachah*, preferably near the place where they will eat.[7] Sephardi women may light there without a *berachah*,[8] or they may light in their room with a *berachah* (as long as nobody has already lit in the room).[9]

When at home for the first Shabbos after birth, the woman should light her own candles, contrary to the custom of years ago when the husband always lit on the first Shabbos.[10]

In many communities it is customary to add an additional candle for every child born.[11]

Kiddush

Kiddush must be made at the Shabbos evening meal, wherever it is being eaten.[12] It is preferable that *kiddush* be made on wine or grape juice. If neither wine nor grape juice is available, *kiddush* should be recited over the challah.[13] First wash *netilas yadayim*, then say the *nussach* of *kiddush*, replacing "*bore peri ha-gafen*" with "*ha-motzi lechem min ha-aretz*."

Two Loaves of Bread   It is preferable to have two whole loaves of bread (challos) or two small rolls at each Shabbos meal. If whole challos are not available, then two slices of bread will fulfill the requirement of *lechem mishneh*.[14] If there is no bread, then one may substitute *mezonos*, such as cake or crackers. When doing this, one should eat at least 6 oz. (170 gr.) of cake or crackers.[15]

If there is no wine, bread or biscuits, one need not go hungry all night or forgo the mitzvah of *oneg Shabbos*, especially not a woman who has just given birth. A woman may, therefore, eat whatever food she has. If she manages to obtain some bread or wine later on, she can recite *kiddush* then.[16]

If she did not hear *kiddush* all night long and wants to eat in the morning, she should recite the regular evening *kiddush* before eating breakfast.

Daytime *kiddush* should be recited over wine or grape juice. If none is available, *kiddush* may be recited over *chamar medinah*,[17] a drink that is not used merely to quench thirst, but is considered of some importance and is used to serve guests.[18] Beer and all hard liquors are considered *chamar medinah*. Many authorities consider coffee, tea, and milk *chamar medinah*,[19] but others say they are not *chamar medinah*.[20] Carbonated drinks and artificial juices are not considered *chamar medinah*,[21] although some authorities maintain that natural juices are considered *chamar medinah*.[22]

Havdalah   In Eretz Yisrael, some hospitals provide a *Havdalah* service for patients. If a woman has missed it, or if her hospital does not provide this service, she can make *Havdalah* by herself.[23] *Havdalah* consists of wine, grape juice or *chamar medinah* (as defined above), spices, a lit

candle and *birkas Havdalah*. Even though women refrain from drinking the *Havdalah* wine when they hear
Havdalah from someone else, the woman reciting
Havdalah for herself must drink the wine at the conclusion of the *birkas Havdalah*.[24]

If a woman has only wine, but no spices or candle,
she should make *Havdalah* on the wine. Later, when she
gets spices and a candle, she can make separate blessings on them.[25] Conversely, if a woman has spices or a
candle, but does not have wine or *chamar medinah* for
Havdalah, she should make separate blessings on either
the spices or the candle, and make *Havdalah* later when
she obtains wine.[26]

It is preferable to make the blessing on a candle
which has at least two wicks (*avukah*). However, if one
has only a one-wick candle, then the *berachah* of *bore
me'orei ha-esh* may be recited over that.[27]

If there is a man present who has already made
Havdalah, a woman should make *Havdalah* for herself
and not be *yotze* with his *Havdalah*.[28] If she has no other
way of hearing *Havdalah*, she may fulfill her obligation
of *Havdalah* by hearing it over the telephone.[29]

Dress

A woman should make an effort to dress nicely on
Shabbos even if she is in the hospital. Wearing a
special Shabbos robe or dress is most appropriate. Our
clothing should not only be pleasing to the eye of our
peers, but should be for the specific purpose of honoring
the Shabbos.[30] Sanctifying the Shabbos in this way will
surely make a woman feel more positive and festive on
this holy day.

NOTES

1. *Shulchan Aruch* 263:6; *Shemiras Shabbos K'hilchasah*, vol. II, 45:6.
2. *Shulchan Aruch*, ibid.; *Mishnah Berurah* 2.
3. *See Responsa, Yechaveh Da'as*, vol. V, 24.
4. *Shulchan Aruch* 263:8.
5. Ibid.
6. Ibid.
7. Ibid.; *Shemiras Shabbos K'hilchasah*, vol. II, 45:6, note 32.
8. *Mishnah Berurah* 2.
9. Ibid.; *Mishnah Berurah* 38.
10. *See* Hebrew appendix.
11. *Otzar Ha-Bris* 5:5.
12. *Shulchan Aruch* 273:1.
13. Ibid. 272:9; *see also Shemiras Shabbos K'hilchasah*, vol. II, 53:15.
14. *Responsa, Mashiv Davar*, ch. 21; *Shemiras Shabbos K'hilchasah*, vol. II, 55:17.
15. *See* R. Zecharyah ben Shelomo, *Hilchos Tzavah*, p. 115.
16. *Shulchan Aruch* 289; *Mishnah Berurah* 10.
17. *Shulchan Aruch* 289:2.
18. *Responsa, Iggros Moshe, Orach Chayim*, vol. II, 75.
19. *Iggros Moshe*, ibid.; *Tzitz Eliezer*, vol. VIII, 16; *Aruch Ha-Shulchan* 296:13.
20. *Responsa, Yechaveh Da'as*, vol. II, 38.
21. *Shemiras Shabbos K'hilchasah*, vol. II, 60:5.
22. *Aruch Ha-Shulchan* 296:13; *Iggros Moshe, Orach Chayim*, vol. II, 75.
23. *Shulchan Aruch* 296:8; *see also Mishnah Berurah*, biur ha-lachah. "Lo yavdel"; *see also Iggros Moshe, Choshen Mishpat*, vol. II, 47:2; *see also Yalkut Yosef*, vol. IV, 296:13; and *see also,* for an alternative opinion, *Shemiras Shabbos K'hilchasah*, vol. II, 61:24, where it says that the woman should make the *berachah* for *ner* after *Havdalah.*
24. *Mishnah Berurah* 296:35; *Yalkut Yosef*, ibid.
25. *Shulchan Aruch* 297:1.
26. Ibid. 298:1.
27. Ibid. 298:2; *see also Mishnah Berurah.*
28. *Mishnah Berurah* 296:36.
29. *Iggros Moshe, Orach Chayim*, vol. IV, 91:4.
30. *Mishnah Berurah* 262:5.

PART THREE:
The Postnatal Phase

16 | The New Mother

The Torah is compared to a woman. Just as a woman comforts her nursing child, so does the Torah comfort all who seek nourishment from her.

MAHARSHA, KIDDUSHIN 2

Labor and delivery are behind you. Now begins your challenging journey on the road to recovery, and the life-long task of raising your child. The fact that Hashem has endowed our bodies with amazing recuperative powers is clearly demonstrated during this postpartum period, also known as the "puerperium." This stage lasts six weeks, during which time your body undergoes many physical changes in an attempt to return to its pre-pregnancy condition.

Uterine Contractions Recovery starts from the moment of birth. Immediately after delivery, the uterus contracts in response to nursing and the administration of oxytocin. These contractions begin the six-week process of involution — the gradual return of the uterus to its original size.

During the first few days following delivery, cramp-like "afterpains" from the contracting uterus can be very uncomfortable. They are especially strong while nursing and become progressively stronger with each succeeding birth. A first-time mother, whose uterus is not as stretched as a multipara's, may not even feel the after-pains. Each day the afterpains decrease in intensity and by the end of the first week they should no longer be felt.

Following both normal and cesarean births, bleed- **Postpartum** ing lasts for approximately six weeks. Postpartum **Bleeding** bleeding (lochia) changes in quantity, color, and consistency throughout this time, as the uterine lining and the placental implantation site undergo repair and regeneration.

The first sequence of bleeding lasts for 3-5 days. It is bright red, with occasional jelled clotting, similar to a menstrual flow.

The second sequence of bleeding continues over the next ten days. Due to the reduced concentration of blood, the discharge is lighter and browner in color.

The third sequence follows from 2-6 weeks postpartum. The discharge is beige with occasional black streaks of old blood.

Continuous heavy bleeding which shows no signs of letting up and the passing of large clots are danger signs. They can indicate that part of the placenta has remained inside the uterus. Bleeding with an offensive odor or fever are signs of infection. If you notice any of these symptoms, you must seek medical attention.

The Torah tells us that a woman is *teme'ah* (ritu- **Niddah** ally impure) for one week after she gives birth to a **Postpartum** boy and for two weeks after the birth of a girl.[1] This *tum'ah* (ritual impurity) has nothing to do with seeing menstrual blood, for even if she did not see blood, she would still be ritually impure for those one or two weeks. Although this is a *chok* — a statute decreed by Hashem without reason or explanation, which must be accepted even though we don't understand it — different explanations have been offered to help us understand the reasons for the mitzvah.

The Kotzker Rebbe quotes the Gemara which teaches us that there are three keys in the sole possession of

Hakadosh Baruch Hu. One of them is the key for a *yoledes,* a woman giving birth. The Divine Presence Itself (*hashra'as Shechinah*) stands by the woman while she gives birth and leaves her after the delivery. It is a rule that whenever the *Shechinah* departs, *tum'ah* takes its place. So, having ended her special relationship with extra *Shechinah* (essentially, *hashgachah peratis* or *hashra'as Shechinah*), the condition of *tum'ah* manifests itself, rendering her ritually impure.[2]

The reason for a two-week period of impurity after the birth of a girl is that giving birth to a daughter — who herself has the potential of giving birth to others — carries with it a much greater sanctity, and subsequently greater impurity.

The Netziv of Volozhin offers an alternative reason. He says that this period of *tum'ah* allows a separation between the husband and wife, so that their marital relationship can resume after a week or two weeks with renewed vigor, as on the day of their marriage.[3]

Since the time of the Talmud, women observe the custom of counting seven clean days after every time they see even a drop of menstrual blood.[4] Therefore, in addition to the seven days for a boy or fourteen days for a girl, women must count seven clean days before going to the *mikveh.* The seven clean days may be counted during the one or two prohibited weeks, provided the woman has stopped bleeding. For instance, if she stopped seeing blood eight days after the birth of her daughter, then she may start counting seven clean days and go to the *mikveh* on the fifteenth day after giving birth, thus fulfilling the fourteen-day prohibition.[5]

Most women continue to see blood for a month to six weeks after giving birth. Nevertheless, once they stop seeing blood, they still must count seven clean days before going to the *mikveh.*

Perineum   The perineum underwent a great deal of stress during delivery. There will be, therefore, soreness and perhaps swelling for the first few postpartum days.

In cases where an episiotomy has been performed, the first three days are the most uncomfortable, but then each succeeding day becomes less painful. If you are in extreme pain, notice redness or swelling around the stitches, or you develop a fever, consult your doctor.

There are several ways to prevent infection and ease the perineal discomfort. Keep the area as clean as possible. At every visit to the bathroom, change your napkin and rinse the area with warm water. A warm sitz bath (a portable basin which fits on a regular toilet seat) three times a day for twenty minutes should also relieve discomfort.

Witch hazel or benzocaine analgesic spray will also be very comforting. Witch hazel pads, available at any pharmacy, are good to bring with you to the hospital as they are helpful in relieving not only perineal discomfort but painful hemorrhoids as well. Remember to wipe from front to back. And, as we mentioned in the prenatal section, taking two warm baths a day is the best way to relieve hemorrhoids.

Sitting on a "doughnut" ring is not recommended as it will only increase swelling. It does not even make it any easier to sit. A soft pillow can serve that purpose.

Episiotomy sutures are made from absorbable material and do not need to be removed. Nevertheless, after one week to ten days you may see some of the black strings of the stitches on your sanitary pad. This is normal and not a cause for alarm.

The episiotomy scar should not interfere with intimate relations. In general, the resumption of intimate relations is not uncomfortable. However, apprehension and exhaustion can have a drying effect upon the natural secretions which lubricate the area. If you have any continuing pain or discomfort, consult your gynecologist.

Fluid Loss

Many women find that they are unusually thirsty during the first week after delivery and they also perspire and urinate more frequently. These symptoms are indicative of the body's reduction of the volume of fluids accumulated during pregnancy. You can expect to lose about 5 lb. (2.5 kg.), in addition to your initial weight loss with delivery, from this release of fluids.[6] Thirst is a natural response to fluid loss, nursing, and deprivation of liquids during labor and delivery. Nursing also causes you to perspire more.

Restricting fluids will not speed weight loss, nor will it prevent breast engorgement. Drink freely! You need plenty of liquids to give you strength and lubricate your bowels.

Early Ambulation and Exercise Most women get out of bed within four hours after delivery. You should *always* be assisted the first time you get out of bed. Every woman can expect to feel dizzy and "wobbly" after delivery. Sit up slowly and dangle your legs at the edge of the bed before standing. The first few times you stand up, you can expect a sudden gush of blood flow, which is a result of the force of gravity.

Your first stop will probably be the bathroom. Have the person assisting you wait nearby until you are comfortably back in bed. The second time up is easier, and you will probably be able to manage on your own.

You will feel better once you are able to go to the bathroom and wash up. At this point you can put on undergarments, a fresh nightgown, and care for yourself. It may be better to wear the hospital's gowns and robes so that your own lingerie won't get soiled.

In general, the hospital staff in the maternity ward allows the woman to do as much as she can for herself. But do not hesitate to be assertive and ask for whatever you need: fresh linen, dressing gowns, maternity pads, breast feeding advice, etc.

If there are no medical contraindications, you may begin postpartum exercises the first day after delivery. During the first few days, exercise, especially walking through the hospital corridors, increases circulation and promotes a feeling of good health. Early ambulation is effective in preventing constipation, the formation of blood clots, and respiratory complications.[7]

Your exercise routine can be intensified as your strength returns. Refer to Chapter 9 on Fitness and Exercise for specific postpartum workouts. Every woman would like to have a flat tummy when she leaves the hospital, but nothing can replace muscle tone. Investing a little time in exercise to tone up our body is far better than borrowing an old girdle or buying an abdominal binder, which will only delay muscle healing.

Preventing Constipation

After delivery, it usually takes a few days to regulate the schedule of bowel movements. If you had an enema before delivery, you will not even need to move your bowels for the first two days. Often the fear of straining stitches or hemorrhoids causes a person to refrain from trying. Inhibiting the urge will only make it more difficult to move your bowels later on. Trying to evacuate will not strain the stitches, and rinsing the area with warm water will relieve any irritation.

A glycerin suppository will lubricate the bowels and prevent straining. Insert the suppository and then lie down for 30 minutes to an hour before going to the bathroom. Glycerin suppositories are available from the maternity ward nurse without a doctor's prescription. Dried fruit, fresh fruits, vegetables and plenty of fluids will also help encourage bowel activity.

Rest

A new mother, or any mother of small children, can never get enough rest. Although the hospital is supposed to be a place for rest and recovery, that's easier said than done. Midnight blood pressure checks, 5:00 A.M. feedings, maintenance workers, doctors' rounds, and visitors all conspire to deprive the new mother of sorely needed rest. However, you can still grab bits of sleep here and there.

Try to pamper yourself and relax as much as you can. Someone else is washing the hospital floor and doing the laundry. Eat and nosh freely without concern for any of the preparation and clean up. Now, no hospital food jokes! Still, it is a good idea to supplement the hospital cuisine with food brought in from home or your favorite restaurant.

Once you are home you will find it difficult to rest, no matter how hard you try. Old and new responsibilities call upon your depleted energy reserves. One of the most practical ways to cope is by lowering your standards and altering your priorities. Don't expect so much of yourself for the first six weeks at least.

Resting after childbirth should not be viewed as spoiling oneself but as a medical imperative. If you are tense and exhausted, you are not the only one who will suffer. Every member of your family, especially the baby, will feel the adverse effects. The rule of thumb is to "sleep when baby sleeps." This may not always be possible, but make sure that you reserve some of baby's sleep periods for your own rest. Housework and other family members can wait a little.

The time to arrange and organize after-birth household help is before the delivery. Family members or hired cleaning help and babysitters should be enlisted. Experienced mothers will advise you that by assuring yourself rest and time to recuperate in the first few weeks, you will return to full functioning capability much sooner than if you try to manage on your own.

Being overtired can lead to neglect of your diet, which will further compound your lack of energy. The postpartum period requires the same wholesome nutrition as pregnancy.

Anemia can also be a cause of tiredness. Hemoglobin is routinely checked the second day after delivery. Supplements may be prescribed by your doctor.

Hormonal Upheaval
A hormone is an organic secretion which acts on specific cells, prompting them to perform particular tasks. Hormones are very powerful, and minute quantities can produce profound effects. Throughout our life cycle, hormones are secreted in varied amounts, inducing diverse bodily reactions. Specific combinations

cause us to ovulate, menstruate, maintain a pregnancy, and lactate.

Immediately after the delivery of the placenta, a woman's hormonal level changes dramatically. Since hormones function in relation to several body processes — growth, temperature, reactions to stress, mood, sleep, and day/night rhythm — we can expect ramifications in any of these areas.

When a woman attributes her distress to hormonal adjustments, she often feels that people are not taking her seriously. She is, however, justified in her complaints to a large degree.

The first few days after delivery are a very emotional time for most women. Estrogen levels are low, and progesterone levels, which were very high during pregnancy, suddenly plummet. Many postpartum women feel the urge to cry or scream. They react emotionally to things that would not normally bother them. This is sometimes referred to as "maternity (postpartum) blues."

While some women have an easy time recovering from the hormonal upheaval of childbirth, others find it overwhelming. When approached with understanding and reassurance, these mood swings usually pass within two weeks after delivery.[8]

There are more extreme, and less common, reactions to the emotional distress of hormonal changes. Postnatal exhaustion and depression and puerperal psychosis have been strongly linked to hormonal and hereditary influences. They are often successfully treated with progesterone supplements.[9]

A routine sixth-week gynecological checkup marks **Sixth-Week** the end of the postpartum period. At that time, **Checkup** your gynecologist will examine the uterus to determine if involution is complete and that everything is healed after the delivery. If you are still staining, the gynecologist will be able to see if the bleeding is coming from the uterus, or perhaps an unhealed cervical or perineal tear. As was mentioned in Chapter 4 on Prenatal

Care, a standard gynecological examination (bi-manual exam and the use of the speculum) does not require you to ask the doctor if he saw blood or to do a *bedikah.*

Daily Drudgery or Inspiration?   The greatest single moment in Jewish history, *Mattan Torah,* is recorded in *Parashas Yisro.* The magnitude of this awesome event caused the souls of all those present to depart from their bodies, and a Divine miracle was necessary to restore them to life.

The most likely follow-up to this special event should have been the building of the *Mishkan* — the Sanctuary, whose purpose was to ensure the Divine Presence among the Jewish People. Yet between the events at Mount Sinai and the building of the Sanctuary, the Torah "interrupts" with *Parashas Mishpatim,* which deals with the laws of buying a slave, thievery, assault, and other mundane facts of life that we hope will not even be relevant to us!

Why was it necessary to disrupt the connection between Mount Sinai and the Sanctuary with these common civil laws? The answer is that Judaism is not like the other "religions." It does not concern itself merely with ritual. By observing the halachic framework of Judaism, we elevate the mundane affairs of our daily lives, and these seemingly routine laws are considered just as holy as any other aspect of Torah. Thus, the penalty incurred by the thief is as important as the law of *tefillin,* or any other ritual. Only when we understand the significance of these laws and observe them properly will we merit the rebuilding of the *Beis Hamikdash* and the Divine Presence among us.

BUILDING A SANCTUARY IN OUR HOME

Having a child is the greatest gift a person can receive. It connects a woman to the Almighty in the same measure as the performance of mitzvos.

First-time mothers look forward to this challenge and view their new role as an expression of loving-kindness, as well as a spiritual goal. However, as time goes on, the tasks involved in caring for a child may seem mundane, boring, and even overwhelming. Changing diapers, feeding, bathing, disciplining, playing in the park, and baking birthday cakes can certainly be tiresome. It may even seem as if these tasks distance us from holiness. After all, raising children takes its toll on one's time and strength and may prevent a woman from attending shul, classes, and even from performing some of the mitzvos with consistency and verve.

But in reality the opposite is true. Although we may not be able to see it in our daily lives, raising children brings us just as close to Hashem as any other mitzvah. In order to reap the rewards of having good children, we must invest a great deal of mundane and repetitive effort in the child's early years.

Just as the Torah mentions the building of the Sanctuary only after the civil laws, so it is with raising children. We must take care of all the child's physical and emotional needs; only then can we bring him up to be a God-fearing Jew. So even though you may not realize it at the time, each action and each chore you invest in raising your child is another step in creating a being who is himself a "holy sanctuary" — a whole new world.

NOTES

1. *Vayikra* 12:1-5.
2. *Amud Ha-Emes, Parashas Tazria.*
3. *Amek Ha-Davar, Parashas Tazria.*
4. *Berachos* 31a.
5. *Shulchan Aruch, Yoreh De'ah* 194:1.
6. A. Pilliteri, *Maternal-Newborn Nursing* (Boston: Little, Brown & Co., 1981), p. 384.
7. M. Myles, *Textbook for Midwives* (Edinburgh: Churchill Livingstone, 1981), p. 450.
8. K. Dalton, *Depression after Birth* (Oxford: Oxford University Press, 1989), p.11.
9. Ibid., p. 124.

17 | Halachic Considerations for the Woman after Childbirth

...So shall you speak to the House of Ya'akov...
SHEMOS 19:3

'The House of Ya'akov' are the women who are swift to perform mitzvos.
SHEMOS RABBAH 28

A woman who has given birth is accorded special consideration with regard to the laws pertaining to Shabbos, Yom Kippur and Tisha B'Av. Her status depends on how much time has elapsed from delivery. For the first seven days, she is considered a *choleh she'yesh bo sakkanah*, a sick person in danger. Within this seven-day period, different laws apply during the first three days and the last four days, which will be discussed in more detail later in this chapter. From the eighth day until the thirtieth day after giving birth, a woman is considered a *choleh she'ein bo sakkanah*, a sick person who is not in danger.

Shabbos *First three days (72 hours)*: If any necessity which is essential to the woman's welfare is perceived, even if she claims she does not need it, one may override the laws of Shabbos in order to provide it for her.[1] However, if both the woman and her doctor claim that it is not a necessity, then one cannot override the laws of Shabbos for her.[2]

If the doctor claims that the woman is not in need but she claims that she is, her wishes are to be fulfilled, for no one knows the extent of the pain or weakness better than the patient herself.[3]

The following are examples of laws which one can override during the first 72 hours:

one may turn on a heater for the patient if she is cold, or a fan or air conditioner if she is suffering from the heat;

if she needs hot food or water and there is none, it is permissible to cook for her;

lights may be turned on and off if necessary.[4]

HOW TO DO THE MELACHAH

It is preferable for a non-Jew to do whatever *melachos* are necessary. However, if a non-Jew is not available, the actions must be performed with a *shinui*. If it is too complicated to do with a *shinui*, it may be performed in its usual manner.[5] Of course, the optimum is to prepare as much as possible before Shabbos.

Fourth day through the seventh day: Although the woman remains in the category of a sick person in danger, we now accept her decision if she claims that she does not need a service which involves overriding the Shabbos laws.[6] However, if her doctor insists that she needs something, it is to be done for her. On the other hand, if her doctor claims she does not need something but she insists that she does, we accede to her request.[7]

Eighth day through the thirtieth day: The woman is considered a sick person who is not in danger. In this situation, a Biblical law (*d'Oraysa*) may be overridden for her by a non-Jew,[8] while an action which involves overriding a Rabbinical law (*d'Rabbanan*) may even be done by a Jew, preferably with a *shinui*.[9] Consult a Rav for further clarification.

If the woman experiences any complication which might be considered dangerous, she reverts to the status of a sick person who is in danger.[10]

Yom Kippur *First three days*: The *halachah* is that the woman does not fast.[11] Therefore, if she feels that she needs to eat regularly, she should do so (without *shiurim*). If her doctor says that she must eat regularly, she should do so.[12]

If the woman is indecisive or silent and does not request either to eat or to fast, there is a difference of opinion about how to handle the situation. Some authorities say that she should eat in a regular manner without *shiurim*,[13] and others say that she should eat with *shiurim*.[14]

If her doctor says she should eat, using *shiurim*, she should use *shiurim*.[15]

If she claims she does not need to eat and her doctor does not disagree, she should nevertheless eat with *shiurim*.[16]

If she feels strong enough to fast and expresses a desire to do so and her doctor says explicitly that she is able to fast, a Rav should be consulted. There are those who say she may fast.[17]

Fourth day through the seventh day: If the woman claims she needs to eat, even if the doctor refutes her, she may eat with *shiurim*.[18]

If she feels that she needs to eat normally or her doctor says she must eat normally, she should do so.[19] If there is no doctor available to determine whether or not she is strong enough to fast, or if the woman is undecided about whether to eat or to fast, then she should eat according to *shiurim*.[20]

If she says she is able to fast and nobody refutes her, then she should fast.[21]

After the seventh day: The new mother is required to fast after the seventh day. However, if she develops complications that make her feel worse and either she or the doctor says she must eat, then she must eat as any sick person who is in danger would.[22]

A woman who has undergone a cesarean section should consult her doctor about her ability to fast, even after the seventh day.[23]

If a woman was told by her doctor to eat or drink —

whether it is in the first seven days, or afterwards due to a complication or weakness — she must obey her doctor's orders. It is clearly forbidden to be *"machmir"* and to fast, for this is not really a *chumrah* in the laws of Yom Kippur, but rather a disregard of the laws which prohibit endangering life (*piku'ach nefesh*).[24]

EATING LESS THAN A SHIUR

A person who is allowed to eat less than a *shiur* should not eat more than 1.1 oz. (30 gr.) of food at intervals of nine minutes. If one feels that nine minutes is too long, then one should make the interval as long as possible, but never less than two minutes between feedings.[25]

The *shiur* for drinking is the volume one can hold in one's cheek, and each person must measure this amount individually. However, the measurement is commonly accepted to be less than 1.4 oz. (40 gr.) for the average person. The same time intervals apply to drinking as apply to eating.[26]

One may eat and drink at the same time because the two actions are considered separately, and the amount of intake is not cumulative with regard to *shiurim.*

It is preferable to prepare the measured portions before Yom Kippur, but if one failed to do so, it is permitted to measure them on Yom Kippur.[27] One can measure in a baby's bottle, which has measurement lines drawn on it. Food which has expanded with air, such as bread and cake, should be compressed before measurement, as the air pockets do not count for the *shiur.*[28]

When one eats less than a *shiur*, she does not have to recite a new *berachah* each time she eats or drinks no matter how long an interval passes between feedings, unless she has taken her mind off the eating and drinking. Also, one should not recite an after-*berachah.*[29]

LAWS FOR YOM KIPPUR

Kiddush is not made, even if Yom Kippur falls on Shabbos. *Lechem mishneh* is not required.

If one eats bread, one must wash *netilas yadayim* as

usual, up to the wrist. *Birkas Ha-mazon* is recited with the addition of "*b'Yom Ha-Kippurim ha-zeh*" in *Ya'aleh v'yavo*. If Yom Kippur falls on Shabbos, one must also add *Retzeh*. However, if one forgot to recite the additions, *Birkas Ha-mazon* is not repeated.[30]

If a woman needs to wash specific areas of her body, she may do so. If she feels that she needs to wear leather shoes, she may do so until the thirtieth day after childbirth.[31]

Tisha B'Av For the first seven days after childbirth a woman does not fast on Tisha B'Av.[32]

She need not fast until after the thirtieth day because during this time she is considered "sick" — a *cholah* — and the Rabbis do not require a sick person to fast on Tisha B'Av.[33] If the woman feels very strong and capable of fasting without undue hardship, she should fast.[34] However, our generation is considered weaker than previous generations, and therefore most women should eat.[35]

Some authorities say that a woman should try to fast for a few hours. If this is too difficult, she should not fast at all.[36] She may eat meat during the Nine Days if she so desires. However, even within thirty days after delivery, it is customary to refrain from eating meat from the seventh of Av, for that is when the *Heichal* was breached.[37]

SYMBOL OF HOPE

The last lamentation said on Tisha B'Av is a *kinah* called "*Alei Tzion v'areha kemo ishah b'tzireha* — Unto Zion and her cities, like a laboring woman." The comparison of *Tzion* to a laboring woman is explained as follows: A woman in labor experiences a great deal of pain, but this pain brings new life into the world. So, too, *Tzion* has suffered so much throughout history, but will soon see new life.

The fetus also struggles through the darkness of the womb, which is called *kever* (grave) in Hebrew. Yet finally it breaks through to a new life in a world of light. So, too, the Jewish People have struggled through the

darkness of exile, which is also called *kever*, and likewise
will break through to a new world of light.
"May You shine a new light on *Tzion* and may we all
speedily merit its light — *Or chadash al Tzion ta'ir;
v'nizkeh chullanu meherah l'oro.*"

NOTES

1. *Shulchan Aruch* 330:4.
2. *Mishnah Berurah* 330:13.
3. Ibid. 330:14.
4. *Shemiras Shabbos K'hilchasah* 32:83; *Toras Ha-Yoledes* 35.
5. *Shemiras Shabbos K'hilchasah* 32, note 220.
6. *Shulchan Aruch* 330:4.
7. *Shemiras Shabbos K'hilchasah* 36:14.
8. *Shulchan Aruch* and *Mishnah Berurah* 330:15, 16.
9. *Shemiras Shabbos K'hilchasah* 36:16, 33:2.
10. *Mishnah Berurah* 330:15; *Sha'ar Ha-Tziyun* 13.
11. *Shulchan Aruch* 617:4.
12. Ibid. 618:1.
13. *Mishnah Berurah* 617:10; *Sha'ar Ha-Tziyun* 12; *biur halachah*
    618, "*K'she'machlin.*"
14. *See* Hebrew appendix.
15. *Shemiras Shabbos K'hilchasah* 39, note 42.
16. *Mishnah Berurah* 617:10; *biur halachah* 618, "*K'shemachlin.*"
17. R. Chayim David Halevi, essay in *Techumin*, vol. IV, 451; *see*
    Hebrew appendix.
18. *Mishnah Berurah* 617:11; *Kaf Ha-Chayim* 617:20; *Shulchan
    Aruch*, Ha-Rav Ba'al Ha-Tanya 617:4.
19. *Kaf Ha-Chayim*, ibid.; *Shemiras Shabbos K'hilchasah* 39:13.
20. *Mishnah Berurah* 617:11; *Sha'ar Ha-Tziyun* 16.
21. *Shemiras Shabbos K'hilchasah* 39:13.
22. *Mishnah Berurah* 617:12.
23. *Kaf Ha-Chayim* 554:28.
24. *Mishnah Berurah* 618:5; *Responsa, Yechaveh Da'as*, vol. I, 61.
25. *Shulchan Aruch* 612:1; *Mishnah Berurah* 618:21; *Shemiras
    Shabbos K'hilchasah* 39:18, note 71.
26. *Shulchan Aruch* 612:9; *Mishnah Berurah* 612:31, 618:7; *Shemi-
    ras Shabbos K'hilchasah* 39:20; *Toras Ha-Yoledes* 52, p. 256.
27. *Sefer Ha-Chinnuch*, mitzvah 313; *Responsa, Yechaveh Da'as*,
    vol. I, 16.

28. *Shemiras Shabbos K'hilchasah* 39:18.
29. Ibid. 39:21.
30. Ibid. 34:31; *Toras Ha-Yoledes* 52:11-14.
31. See note 30.
32. *Eliyahu Rabbah* 554:8; *Kaf Ha-Chayim* 554:36.
33. *Shulchan Aruch* 554:6.
34. Rama and *Mishnah Berurah* 554:12; Maharshal 53.
35. *See* Hebrew appendix.
36. *See* Hebrew appendix.
37. *Magen Avraham* 554:9.

18 | Birkas Ha-gomel

Birkas Ha-gomel was established in place
of the thanksgiving offering.

ROSH, BERACHOS, ch. 9

All of the sacrifices were brought for sins
except for the thanksgiving offering, which
was brought for a miracle. Hakadosh
Baruch Hu said: 'This is more beloved to
me than all the other sacrifices.'

MIDRASH TANCHUMA 13:7

It is customary for the mother to say *Birkas Ha-gomel* after giving birth. This *berachah* should not be recited until after she feels strong, at least seven days after
delivery.[1] However, she should not wait longer than
thirty days after she feels strong.[2]

The blessing should be recited in the presence of a
minyan of ten men. Considering that "the honor of a
woman is in her modesty," she should say it from the
women's section of the synagogue, behind the *mechitzah*
(separation). When *Birkas Ha-gomel* is said at home, the
woman should stand at the entrance to the room the
men are in, as a substitute for a *mechitzah*, but if the
men are closely related to her, she may recite the *berachah* in their presence.[3]

It is preferable for the blessing to be recited during
the daytime. However, if the mother has already said the
blessing at night, the mitzvah is still considered fulfilled.[4] Some authorities rule that there is no problem

whatsoever if the woman recited the blessing at night, and in many places it is the custom to gather ten men in the home of the new mother on *motza'ei Shabbos* or any other night to enable her to say the blessing in the presence of a minyan.[5]

The *berachah* should be recited while standing, but those listening should sit.[6]

If a woman feels uncomfortable saying the blessing before a quorum of ten men, a Rav should be consulted for alternative possibilities.[7]

NOTES

1. *Shulchan Aruch* 219:1; *Mishnah Berurah* 2; *Kaf Ha-Chayim* 219:7.
2. *Mishnah Berurah* 219:8; see *Toras Ha-Yoledes* 62:5, which brings the opinion that only from 30 days after giving birth can a woman say the *berachah*; see R. Nissim Sasson, *Todas Chayim*, p. 78, where the author writes that if the woman still feels weak, she must wait until she feels stronger, and then say the *berachah.*
3. *Kaf Ha-Chayim* 219:3; see *Responsa, Yechaveh Da'as*, vol. IV, 16.
4. *Responsa, Chasam Sofer, Orach Chayim* 51; *Kaf Ha-Chayim* 219:14; Ben Ish Chai, first year, *Parashas Ekev:* 3.
5. *Responsa, Tzitz Eliezer*, vol. XIII, 17.
6. Ben Ish Chai, first year, *Parashas Ekev:* 3; *Mishnah Berurah* 219:4.
7. *See* Hebrew appendix.

19 | The Newborn

Out of the mouths of babes and sucklings
You have founded strength.
TEHILLIM 8:3

The first weeks after delivery can be defined most accurately as a whirlwind of activity. It's not just "*mazal tovs*" and presents. The newborn himself undergoes a tremendous adjustment to life outside the womb, while the new mother — and a woman is a new mother with every birth — has to recuperate and restructure her life and activities around her new baby. Family members open their hearts to welcome the new addition, with each one making significant personal adjustments. It is the mother, however, who has the overall responsibility for the wellbeing of the entire family. She must make sure that each family member adjusts properly and, most importantly, that she and the baby receive the care they require.

Your Newborn's Needs

Baby has finally arrived. *Mazal tov!* "Now what do I do!?" Not only do first-time mothers ask this question, but even veteran mothers experience new challenges and responsibilities with each newborn.

It is important to realize that no one else can take care of your baby like you can. If the baby was not "rooming-in" with you in the hospital, then coming home with your newborn will be your first opportunity to fully assume your role as mother.

There are supplies your baby needs for his trip home. You should arrange to have the following items brought to the hospital the day before discharge:

T-shirt	receiving blanket
baby sleeper (stretchy/Babygro)	two diapers

In winter, add another warm outfit over the baby sleeper, and protect the baby's head with a hat. Make sure your baby is secure in an infant car seat during his first journey in a car.

Customs differ as to when to acquire baby furniture and a carriage. Some people buy baby items only after the birth. Others may place an order at a baby specialty store, with the proviso that their purchases will be delivered only after the baby is born. In households where there is already a child (children), the new baby may receive almost everything he needs second-hand from his generous sibling(s). Whatever the source of baby's needs, preparing the hand-me-downs, choosing new items, and receiving gifts are great fun. Enjoy!

The following is a list of items which should always be on hand for the newborn:

diapers	pacifiers, bottles (if necessary)
baby wipes	electronic (digital) thermometer
baby ointment	standard thermometer
baby powder	cotton swabs (Q-tips)
cotton balls	soapless soap (liquid)
70% alcohol	nasal aspirator
baby oil	small medicine bottle with dropper
baby lotion	

Weight   During the first year of life, weight measurement is an important tool to assess baby's well-being and growth. The newborn is weighed immediately upon delivery and daily thereafter as long as he is hospitalized. During the first few days, a baby usually loses 5-10% of his birth weight due to fluid loss. However, within ten

CONVERSION OF BABIES' WEIGHTS (lb./oz. to gr.)

lb. \ oz.	0	1	2	3	4	5	6	7	8	9	10	11	12	13	14	15
0		28	57	85	113	142	170	198	227	255	283	312	340	368	397	425
1	454	482	510	539	567	595	624	652	680	709	737	765	794	822	850	879
2	907	935	964	992	1020	1049	1077	1105	1134	1162	1190	1219	1247	1275	1304	1332
3	1360	1389	1418	1446	1475	1503	1531	1560	1588	1616	1645	1673	1701	1730	1758	1786
4	1815	1843	1871	1900	1928	1956	1985	2013	2041	2070	2098	2126	2155	2183	2211	2240
5	2268	2296	2325	2353	2381	2410	2438	2466	2495	2523	2551	2580	2608	2636	2655	2683
6	2721	2750	2778	2806	2835	2863	2891	2920	2948	2976	3005	3033	3061	3090	3118	3146
7	3175	3203	3231	3260	3258	3316	3345	3373	3401	3430	3458	3486	3515	3543	3571	3600
8	3628	3656	3685	3713	3741	3770	3798	3826	3855	3883	3911	3940	3968	3996	4025	4053
9	4081	4110	4138	4166	4195	4223	4251	4280	4308	4336	4355	4383	4421	4450	4468	4506
10	4535	4563	4591	4620	4648	4676	4705	4733	4761	4790	4818	4846	4875	4903	4931	4960

days following delivery he will have regained his birth weight and often surpasses it.

In some cases when adequate breast milk supply is in doubt, a baby is checked to see if he is receiving enough. This is called a weighing trial. The infant is weighed, nursed, and then weighed again. A weight gain of at least 1.75 oz. (50 gr.) demonstrates that the baby is receiving an adequate amount of breast milk.

During the first year, a newborn is routinely weighed once a month.

Temperature   Immediately after birth, the newborn's temperature will be taken rectally. There are two reasons for this: to measure body temperature, and to make sure there is a patency (an opening) from the anus to the rectum. Thereafter, as long as the infant is in the hospital, temperature will be measured once a day, using the axillary (under the arm) method.

During the first 8-12 hours after birth, the newborn is placed in a special observation area, which is kept at a higher temperature than the rest of the nursery. Since the temperature-regulating mechanism of the newborn is still immature, the infant is especially vulnerable to temperature extremes immediately after birth.

At home, you will have the responsibility of providing sufficient heat for your baby. But it's important not to overdo it, for although your baby needs to be kept warm, he can become uncomfortable and sweat if kept *too* warm.

If the bathroom or bedroom cannot be adequately heated, avoid the temptation to give your baby a long, luxurious bath. When the baby becomes soiled, just wash off the diaper area as quickly as possible under the tap. A bath is nice — but not at the expense of baby's health.

Techniques to Measure Temperature   Temperature is taken rectally until one year of age. An electronic thermometer is quick and accurate, but you will also need a regular thermometer for Shabbos. A standard thermometer will take about two to three minutes to reach the correct reading.

The tip of the thermometer may be lubricated with a little petroleum jelly. This makes insertion easier for you and more comfortable for the baby. Lay the baby on his stomach on your lap or bed. Insert the tip of the thermometer so that it lightly touches the inner wall of the anus. Gently press the buttocks together with one hand and hold the legs still with the other. The baby can also lie on his side.

Centigrade-Fahrenheit Equivalents	
Centigrade	Fahrenheit
41	106
40	104
39	102
38	100.4
37 (normal body temp.)	98.6
36	97

To convert Centigrade to Fahrenheit:
$$°F = (°C \times 9/5) + 32$$

To convert Fahrenheit to Centigrade:
$$°C = (°F - 32) \times 5/9$$

The child from one year to about six years old may experience less trauma when an axillary temperature is taken. It takes about four to eleven minutes to achieve an accurate axillary reading, while it takes about three minutes to measure temperature orally. Oral temperature measurement is only recommended after six years of age.

Again, don't overdo it. Infants do not generally enjoy the experience of measuring temperature, and they naturally heat up when crying. Baby's temperature should be taken only if you really suspect an illness with fever.

Sleep

During the first few weeks of life, your baby may sleep 16-20 hours out of every 24. Some babies seem to sleep from feeding to feeding. Sleeping patterns vary depending on the activity and temperament of the baby.

Since newborns do not differentiate between night and day, it is up to you to regulate their day accordingly. One way is not to allow your baby to sleep more than 3-4 hours at a time during the day. Then he will soon become accustomed to longer sleep periods at night. Also, it is not always necessary to feed the baby each time he wakes at night, especially if he awakens more often than once every three hours. Sometimes simply giving a pacifier or rocking the cradle or carriage will be sufficient to soothe the baby back to sleep.

It's good to alternate your baby's sleeping positions. According to the World Health Organization's (W.H.O.) recommendation, which has been adopted worldwide, infants should be placed on their back rather than on their stomachs to sleep. This is thought to help prevent S.I.D.S. (Sudden Infant Death Syndrome), which is believed to be caused by suffocation. There is no cause for worry that a baby might spit up and choke while sleeping on his back, according to pediatricians. Baby may also sleep comfortably and safely on his side.

Feeding Patterns
Feeding schedules at the hospital may be inflexible, firmly established routines. Many mothers feel some concern about this. If you feel it is important, discuss your feelings with hospital personnel before choosing where to give birth; and after you give birth, tell them about any special care instructions you have in mind for the baby.

You may start to breast feed your newborn immediately after delivery, though many hospitals will still offer sterile water a few hours after birth to determine if the esophagus is properly formed.

Hospitals usually provide feedings on a schedule of every 3-4 hours. In many instances the nurses give the babies their midnight feeding, enabling you to catch up on rest and sleep through the night. If you want to give your baby his nighttime feeding, you should arrange this with the nursery staff.

"Rooming-in" is a popular option which allows mother and baby to be together continuously. The mother provides the bulk of the baby's care (with a little help from the nurses).

In most cases your hospital stay will be for only 2 1/2 days, so any hospital routines will not have long-term ramifications. Once you are home, you will be able to make your own decisions about the feeding schedule.

Following delivery, the remaining part of the um- **Umbilical**
bilical cord is white, translucent and smooth. With **Cord Care**
each day, the cord stump degenerates, becoming
black, dried and shriveled. Dab the area with a cotton
ball soaked in 70% alcohol, making sure to reach the
area under the cord. The cord will fall off 7-10 days after
the birth. Don't be surprised if the stump detaches itself
during your gentle cleaning treatments or if you just find
it in the diaper. Continue to apply alcohol locally for another few days until the area heals completely. Do not
totally immerse your baby's body in water until the cord
falls off.

What your baby eats will influence the appearance, **Excretion**
consistency and frequency of bowel movements.
During the first day or two of life, all newborns pass meconium, a stool which is blackish-green and sticky.

On the second or third day of life, the newborn's stool
will be green and loose. This is called transitional stool.

By the fourth day, a breast-fed infant will pass 3-4
light yellow stools per day. The stool of breast-fed babies
is generally loose, which should not be confused with diarrhea. It is also not uncommon for babies to pass as
many as six bowel movements a day. An infant fed with
formula usually passes 2-3 bright yellow stools per day.
His stool will have more form and a stronger odor than
the stool of breast-fed infants.

Constipation is rare in breast-fed infants, but may be
experienced by bottle-fed infants. It is attributed to insufficient fluid intake, inaccurate use of formula, or an
incompatibility with the formula in use.

Colic is a general term referring to newborn abdominal pain of unknown origin. Some of the projected
causes are: overfeeding, not "burping" the baby, the
wrong formula, too much air in the bottle, or a nervous
mother. Since a definitive diagnosis cannot be made,
colic is often defined simply as a "fussy period." It occurs
most frequently in the evening hours and may keep new
parents pacing the floors or taking late evening strolls

seeking comfort for the baby. To release trapped gas, it may be helpful to change the baby's position and place him on his stomach, or over your shoulder, or do knee-chest exercises with him. Many couples have found that carrying baby around in a "Snuggli" baby carrier will quiet his cries.

Colic miraculously disappears around three months of age, so the tired mother can look forward to eventual relief.

Diaper
Change   The infant is often stimulated to move his bowels during a feeding. Of course, this usually happens right after you have put a fresh diaper on him! Don't despair. As time passes, you will become familiar with the baby's schedule and be able to anticipate the best time to change him. A possible option is to nurse from one side, then burp the baby and change his diaper. Afterwards, the baby will generally fall asleep with a clean diaper while nursing from the second side.

The best way to clean baby's bottom after a bowel movement is under the tap with warm water and liquid soap. Disposable wipes are filled with chemicals that may cause irritation, so use them only when traveling. Ointment or powder need be applied only in case of irritation. On Shabbos or *Yom Tov*, you should limit yourself to powder, but ointment can be used if it has been spread on a gauze pad before Shabbos. The pad can then be positioned on the diaper area without any attempt to distribute it over the skin.[1]

Diapers:
Cloth or
Disposable   If cloth diapers are used, it is best to start with at least two dozen. Soiled diapers should be soaked in a large, lidded bucket which has been filled halfway with a solution of water, half a cup of detergent, and a quarter cup of bleach. This method is forbidden on Shabbos and *Yom Tov*, when soiled diapers should be stored in a dry bucket or bag. Many cloth-diaper users prefer the convenience of using disposable diapers on Shabbos (consult your Rav) or when traveling.

Although disposable diapers are more costly, they save time and energy. When the baby begins to eat solid food, his bowel movements will resemble those of an adult. In order to prevent the odor from pervading the house, seal offensive diapers in a plastic bag before placing them in the waste bin. But even if you will be using only disposable diapers on the baby's bottom, you will still find it convenient to have a number of cloth diapers on hand for other purposes.

Skin Care

Infant skin care involves a varied treatment in response to baby's delicate skin. Most minor skin ailments can be prevented by using a mild soap and keeping baby dry and clean.

A baby's skin is equipped to moisturize itself, so it is a good idea to avoid the overuse of skin care products. Baby lotion should be used only if the baby has dry skin, and then sparingly.

Some babies have little pimples on their cheeks ("baby acne"). Although this condition may last several months, it will eventually disappear by itself, and no extra care is necessary. You could try switching to a milder laundry detergent or fabric softener, as the condition may be due to the baby's sensitivity to some of the ingredients in your regular laundry products. The baby's face should be washed as usual.

"Cradle cap" (seborrheic dermatitis) on baby's scalp should be treated with baby oil applied to the crusty patches for several days, and then by gently combing and shampooing to remove the crust.

Stuffy Nose

Some newborns snort and snore when they breathe and sleep as if they had a cold, but it is only due to the retention of mucus in the upper respiratory tract. Unless accompanied by coughing, watery eyes and large quantities of mucus, it is not a cold.

This condition is uncomfortable for the baby, and can be alarming for the new mother. Treatment with saline nose drops will help clear the stuffy nose. The drops may cause the baby to sneeze (thus clearing out the nasal passage), but at the very least he will be able to feed more easily. Saline drops can be purchased at the pharmacy or made at home:

SALINE DROPS RECIPE:
Take one cup of boiled water (cooled, of course).
Add one teaspoon of salt.
Mix and pour into medicine bottle with dropper.
Squirt twice into each nostril before each feeding.

For stuffiness which is extra-stubborn, replace the teaspoon of salt with half a teaspoon of salt and half a teaspoon of baking soda. Change the saline solution once a week.

In addition to the saline drops, use a nasal aspirator to suction out the mucus which can be seen at the edge of the nostrils. First squeeze the bulb of the aspirator and then gently insert the tip into the nostril. When the bulb is released, the mucus will be sucked into the aspirator. The aspirator must be cleaned with soap and water after each use.

If the baby is having difficulty sleeping because of nasal congestion or a real cold, raise the head of his bed to a 20-30° angle by placing a towel or blanket under the mattress. Just as sleeping with an extra pillow helps the adult to breathe better, elevating the baby's head will help him breathe better. If the baby has fever, or if his stuffiness persists, he may have a cold. The pediatrician should be consulted.

Eye Color   It is a common myth that all newborns have blue eyes. In fact, some infant eyes are tinged with gray or brown. By three months you should notice the shade of baby's eyes becoming a more definitive color, and by six months the eye color is stable.

Medical Care   Every newborn is thoroughly examined on the day of birth and on the day of discharge from the hospital. Heart rate, respiration and overall appearance are scrutinized. Neuromuscular function is tested by observing certain reflexes which demonstrate neurological maturity and well-being, such as:

Moro Reflex. When an infant is startled by a sudden loud noise or movement, he throws his arms out and pulls his legs up as if to ward off an attacker. This reflex disappears at the end of the fourth month, when the infant can roll away from danger.

Rooting Response. Stroking an infant's cheek will cause him to turn his head to that side and search for his mother's breast. This reflex also disappears when it is no longer needed — about the sixth week of life, when the eyes can focus steadily and the food source can be identified.

Grasp Response. The baby will firmly grasp a finger placed in the palm of his hand. This reflex disappears between six weeks to three months after birth, when babies begin to grasp meaningfully.

Step-in-Place Reflex. When the baby is held in a standing position with his feet on a flat surface, he will make stepping movements. This reflex disappears by three months of age. At four months, the baby can bear a good portion of his weight and will not need to make the stepping movements.

In addition to this impressive array of reflexes, the newborn is equipped with many special senses:

Hearing. Within hours after birth, the amniotic fluid drains from the middle ear and the newborn will be able to hear.[2] If he is actively crying and a bell is rung, he will stop crying and seem to listen. He will also become calm in response to a soothing or motherly voice and be startled by loud noises. Standard hearing assessment is done between seven and nine months.

Sight. Newborns see as soon as they are born, and it is believed that they might even have this ability in utero.[3] The newborn demonstrates sight at birth by blinking at strong light. He cannot, however, follow objects past the midline of vision and easily loses track of things. A newborn's vision becomes more accurate at six to eight weeks and at three months he can follow past midline.

Touch. The sense of touch is well-developed at birth. An infant will become quiet in response to a gentle touch. He will also react to painful stimuli.

Taste. Research has shown that a newborn has discriminating taste buds, which function even prior to birth. An infant will turn away from a bitter taste, but readily accept the sweet taste of milk or sugared water.[4]

Smell. As soon as the nose is clear of mucus and amniotic fluid, the newborn can smell. He recognizes his mother's breast as a food source in part by smelling the breast milk.

First Impressions A newborn's head is disproportionately large in comparison to his body. In addition to the head taking up about one-fourth of the infant's total length, it has also undergone "molding" during the birth process — adapting itself to fit the contours of the mother's pelvis and birth canal. The head may, therefore, appear too long, squashed, or even a bit bent out of shape. Within a few days, however, it will return to a normal configuration.

FONTANELLES

Fontanelles are the spaces or openings where the skull bones join together. At the top of the baby's head, toward the front, is the soft spot known as the "anterior fontanelle." When this diamond-shaped cleft appears indented, it might be a sign of dehydration. On the other hand, it may protrude in response to crying or straining, or as a result of increased intracranial pressure. The anterior fontanelle closes at 12-18 months of age.

The "posterior fontanelle" is a triangular space toward the back of the head. Less significance is attributed to this soft spot because it remains open for only a short time, closing by the end of the second month.

Baby's First Blood Test Before the newborn is discharged from the hospital, his blood will be tested to determine blood type and Rh factor, and to screen for PKU. PKU (phenylketonuria) is the lack of the enzyme necessary to metabolize phenylalanine, an amino acid found in milk and artificial sweeteners. One out of 7,500 newborns are born with this deficiency, which can cause mental retardation if undetected. The treatment for PKU is a diet low in phenylalanine.

In addition to PKU, infants of Sephardic lineage will often be tested for G6-PD, a recessive disease found among Sephardic Jews and non-Jews of Mediterranean descent. G6-PD (glucose 6 — phosphate dehydrogenase deficiency) causes the breakdown of blood cells in children or adults who ingest fava beans or drugs such as aspirin (Optalgin). If either parent has G6-PD, or a family relative suffers from it, the newborn will be tested for this deficiency.

Baby's First Medical Records

Upon leaving the hospital, you will receive two copies of the discharge letter. One is for your own personal records, and the other is for your baby's medical file. Bring this letter along to your baby's first checkup, ten days after birth.

NOTES

1. *Shulchan Aruch* 328:22.
2. A. Pilliteri, *Maternal-Newborn Nursing* (Boston: Little, Brown & Co., 1981), p. 428.
3. Ibid., and *Yoma* 82. The Gemara supports the idea of the fetus sensing things outside the womb, specifically that the fetus smells a scent and has a desire for it.
4. F. Caplan, *The First Twelve Months of Life* (New York: Bantam Books, 1983), p. 14.

20 | It's a Boy!

*The glory of sons are fathers, the glory of
fathers are sons.*
BERESHIS RABBAH 63:2

Mazal tov — a son is born — a son who will, with God's
help, be a source of pride and joy to his family and the
entire Jewish People. Along with the birth of a son come
many *simchahs*, and several customs, the greatest *simchah* being, of course, the bris (*bris milah*). For a firstborn son, there is also, possibly, a *pidyon ha-ben*
(consult your Rav to find out if this applies to your son).

Shema Yisrael During the first week of the baby's birth, prior to
the bris, it is customary in some communities that
children come to the house of the newborn and recite the
words of *Shema Yisrael* in his presence. The *Zohar* explains that before the bris, impure spiritual forces try to
harm the infant; therefore, children who are too young to
have sinned come and recite *Shema Yisrael*, the prayer
which has the power to keep these harmful forces away
from the newborn. We give the children sweets in order
to encourage them to come.[1]
The significance of this custom is expressed once
again at the opening of the bris ceremony in Eretz Yisrael, as the father declares, "*Shema Yisrael, Hashem
Elokeinu, Hashem Echad.*" But why the *Shema*? Why say

the *Shema* to an infant who has no understanding or awareness of what is happening to him?

Although the source of this custom is kabbalistic, we can still appreciate its significance, make it a part of our everyday lives, and also transmit it to our children.

Shema Yisrael: The Ultimate Declaration

Rabbi Yehoshua ben Korchah asked: "Why does *Kerias Shema* open with *Shema Yisrael* followed by *V'hayah im shamo'a?*" He answers: So that we should accept the yoke of the Heavenly Kingdom and then accept the yoke of mitzvos.[2]

The recitation of *Shema Yisrael* is our acceptance of the yoke of Heaven. *Chazal* tell us that the complete *Kerias Shema* includes the Ten Commandments.[3] But even the first verse alone incorporates the major precepts of Judaism. By saying the *Shema*, we acknowledge the existence of God and affirm that He is One. We express our connection to *Am Yisrael* and declare our belief that in the future the whole world will acknowledge the Kingdom of Heaven. Expressing this faith is *Kiddush Hashem*, the sanctification of God's Holy Name — the purpose of our existence.

Shema Yisrael Throughout History

The Torah records Moshe *Rabbenu* as being the first to say the *Shema* in his "farewell address" to the Jewish People.[4]

The Gemara maintains that the twelve sons of Ya'akov actually preceded Moshe in saying it. When Ya'akov was about to reveal the end of days to his children, he was concerned that one of them might be a non-believer. His sons reassured him immediately and cried out, "*Shema Yisrael, Hashem Elokeinu, Hashem Echad.*"[5]

Chazal tell us that, even before this, Ya'akov himself recited *Kerias Shema*. After a twenty-two-year separation from his son Yosef, he finally went down to *Mitzrayim* to see him. As Yosef came to greet him, he collapsed on his father's shoulder and cried. But the Torah does not say that Ya'akov did the same. Why not? Rashi (citing *Chazal*) explains that Ya'akov was saying *Kerias Shema*.[6]

But the great emotional and historical significance of the *Shema* does not derive from Moshe *Rabbenu*, or from the twelve sons of Ya'akov, or even from Ya'akov himself, whose lifelong hope was that his descendants recite the *Shema* twice daily (*Pesikta Rabbati* 31), but rather from Rabbi Akiva, who sacrificed his life in order to teach Torah. Subjected to horrendous torture by the Roman executioner, he told his disciples that it had been his lifelong wish to demonstrate his complete faith in the Almighty. With his dying breath, he sanctified God's Name, crying out: "*Shema Yisrael, Hashem Elokeinu, Hashem Echad,*" and as he finished saying "*Echad,*" his soul departed.[7]

The cry of *Shema* has always symbolized the ultimate manifestation of faith in the gravest situations. Countless Jews throughout the ages have bravely died *al Kiddush Hashem* with these sacred words on their lips. The learned, the layman, old and young, the believer and even those who claimed to be non-believers, have left this world emulating Rabbi Akiva.

A PERSONAL ACCOUNT

In the summer of 1982 (during Israel's war in Lebanon) a young soldier from Haifa lay in a hospital bed in Jerusalem's Hadassah Hospital. His hands and body were covered with wounds and burns; his shoulder, jaw and teeth were broken; even his tongue had been stitched up. He had lost some vision in one eye, and specks of shrapnel still dotted his face. Doctors from every department were involved in his treatment.

He told the following story:

> It was the first day of the war, and I was serving in the IDF's Nachal infantry unit. We had just entered the city of Tzur (Tyre). I was seated in the armored personnel carrier near the field radio. It was hot and I was sweating profusely. I took off my protective goggles to wipe my eyes from the perspiration. I took off my fire-resistant gloves too. Just as I removed the goggles, an enemy RPG [rocket-propelled grenade] ripped into our vehicle. It struck the

communication box and it hit me in the face, smashing my jaw and teeth. Everyone jumped out. I was the only one left. I knew that in only a few seconds the whole vehicle, with all of our own ammunition in it, would explode, so I tried desperately to pull myself out. I couldn't. I tried again but had no strength to move. I was sure that my life was over.

Although I was born and raised in Israel, I never had a religious education, never walked into a synagogue, never even prayed. But I was certain that this was the end for me, so for the first time in my life I said, "*Shema Yisrael, Hashem Elokeinu, Hashem Echad.*" Just as I said "*Echad,*" I felt someone grab me under my arms and yank me out, only a fraction of a second before the vehicle blew up.[8]

Faith Beyond Understanding

We mentioned earlier that first we accept the yoke of Heaven and only afterwards accept the yoke of mitzvos. This is because many mitzvos are logical and we might very well observe them even without a commandment from God. We accept the Heavenly yoke first in order to proclaim that we accept responsibility for observing all our mitzvos *because* they are the commandments of our Creator.[9]

That proclamation also gives us strength to accept the mitzvos that we do not understand, for while many of Hashem's mitzvos are logical, some seem to be completely illogical. Similarly, many events occurring in the world encourage and strengthen our belief, yet many events in our personal lives and throughout history make it harder to believe. Therefore, we say *Shema Yisrael* in the daytime, when everything is clear and bright and we understand the way of God. And we also say *Shema Yisrael* at night, when life is dark and unclear and we do not understand the ways of God.

When a child is born, other children come over to the house and say *Shema Yisrael,* even though the newborn cannot understand. This act symbolizes the expression of pure belief that goes beyond understanding. The "impure spiritual forces" that threaten to harm the newborn may cause not physical harm, but rather spiritual harm. They might, for example, influence him to be more materialistic or rebellious when he grows up. *Shema Yisrael,* as the Netziv of Volozhin says, has the power to bring one to loftier, more spiritual pursuits in life.[10] Reciting *Shema* to a newborn can strengthen him to have greater potential for spirituality. After the bris, he bears on his body that symbol of faith, but before the bris, he needs the expression of belief that connects him with Hashem. The fact that he does not understand is not important, because belief is above our understanding.

It is this faith, imbedded in the soul of every Jew, that made a little boy of the age of three named Avram seek God. It is this faith that we try to instill in all of our children.

Other Halachos and Customs The night before the bris, it is customary to learn Torah in the house of the infant,[11] but customs differ as to what is learned and how the occasion is celebrated. It is appropriate to follow the customs of one's community.

It is a common Ashkenazic custom to hold a *Shalom Zachar* on the first Friday night after the baby's birth at the home of the newborn. Light refreshments, including *arbes* (chickpeas) are served (but not a full meal).[12] One of the reasons given for this custom is that the guests come to comfort the newborn as he is mourning for the Torah that he forgot upon leaving his mother's womb.[13]

There are a number of English-language books available on the *halachos* and customs of *bris milah,* and it is highly recommended that new parents familiarize themselves with the pertinent information in advance of the ceremony. Here are a few points to consider that might help make the bris go more smoothly:

In Ashkenazic communities it is deemed a great honor to take part in the bris. The various "tasks" involved are therefore given out as "*kibbudim*" — honors — to some of the guests.

The *kibbudim* are:

1. *Kvater* and *kvaterin* — usually a married couple. Preferably, this couple has not yet had children of their own, as the honor is considered a "*segullah*" (a good omen) to have children. The baby's mother hands the child over to the *kvaterin*, who passes him to her husband, the *kvater*. He brings the baby into the room where the bris is to take place.

2. *El ha-kise shel Eliyahu:* The honoree's task is to place the newborn on the *kise shel Eliyahu* — the elevated, often ornate "throne of Elijah," for tradition says that Elijah attends every bris. (If necessary, one may add other guests for this honor, as one guest may hand the baby to the next honoree.)

3. *Me-ha-kise shel Eliyahu:* The honor of taking the baby from the "throne."

4. *Sandak:* This is the highest honor, usually given to the grandfather, an elder, or a great scholar. The honoree holds the newborn across his knees while the bris is being performed, an honor considered equal to offering up the holy incense in the *Beis Hamikdash.*

5. *Mohel:* The mohel should be God-fearing and proffessionally competent.

6. *Amidah la-berachos:* The honoree holds the baby while the *berachah* of "*Asher kiddesh yedid mi-beten*" is recited.

7. *Berachos:* The honoree recites the *berachah* of "*Asher kiddesh yedid mi-beten*" and names the baby. (See Chapter 22 on Naming Your Child.)

It is best to bring at least three *tallisos* (prayer shawls) to the bris, for the custom is that all the honorees wear a *tallis.*

Every *mohel* gives his own specific care instructions. **Bris Milah** He will usually visit you a day or two before the bris to examine the baby and let you know what you need for the bris. It is usually recommended that the baby not be fed for an hour prior to the bris.

Care for the Bris Milah After the bris, you will want to feed your son to calm him, though he may already be drowsy from the wine given him during the bris.

About half an hour after the bris, the *mohel* will once again examine the baby to ensure that there is no excess bleeding. He may give you an antiseptic powder or solution to apply to the wound. Do not use this preparation on the area of the umbilical cord. Continue umbilical care as previously described. It is important that the baby continue to urinate as usual. Expect your baby to be a bit fussy for the first 24 hours after the bris.

The day after the bris, the *mohel* will visit your baby again. Follow his instructions, and make sure to keep the site clean. The bris appears red and sore with a thin yellow film over the surface, similar to a scab. Don't try to wash it away. The bris heals very quickly, and the baby is usually allowed to receive a regular bath on the third or fourth day after the bris.

The baby may be uncomfortable sleeping on his stomach after the bris. Put him to sleep on his side for 3-4 days until he can again comfortably sleep on his stomach.

Special Bris Considerations It is every parent's wish to fulfill the mitzvah of *bris milah* at the proper time — *b'ito u'vi-zemano* — that is, on the eighth day. However, the newborn's health is always taken into consideration. Sometimes the bris must be postponed. The following are some of the *halachos* which apply to postponing the bris:

SICKNESS

If a newborn was sick, the *bris milah* may not be performed until seven days after the baby is considered healthy.[14] For example, if a newborn was put into an incubator because he could not maintain a stable body temperature, we must wait seven days from when the baby was removed from the incubator before the bris may be performed — even if the doctor says that it may be performed before that time.[15] If the baby had a fever of 100.4°F (38°C) or higher, we must wait seven days from the time the temperature returned to normal. However, if the fever was caused by slight dehydration, which is very easily cured, then we may do the bris when the doctor permits it.[16]

THE NEWBORN'S SIZE

There are some doctors who are of the opinion that a newborn who weighs less than 5.9 lb. (2.7 kg.) should not be circumcised. *Chazal*, however, never consider size as a factor in deferring a bris. Therefore, as soon as the baby reaches a weight deemed adequate by his doctor, the bris may be performed immediately, without waiting seven days.[17] According to Dr. Matityahu Erlichman, pediatric specialist and attending physician at Jerusalem's Shaare Zedek Hospital, there is no need to wait for the baby to reach a certain weight. Even a baby whose birth weight was 4.6 lb. (2.1 kg.), who is eating regularly and gaining weight, can have a bris on schedule. On the other hand, if a baby was born weighing 6.6 lb. (3 kg.) but is losing weight, this may be considered a sign of illness and requires medical examination, and the bris may be postponed for seven days from the time the baby begins to gain weight.

JAUNDICE

If, on the day of the bris, the newborn has jaundice, the bris is delayed.[18]

Jaundice manifests itself as a yellowish tint in the skin and sclera (the "whites") of the eyes. Every fetus is endowed with a high red blood cell count to supply the huge amounts of oxygen necessary in utero. After birth, these excess red blood cells are broken down and excreted from the body through the feces. Approximately half of all newborns have difficulty excreting the end product of red blood cell breakdown. As a result, excess bilirubin remains in the body and permeates the skin, giving it a yellow tinge.

Jaundice usually appears by the second or third day

after birth. If it is suspected, a blood test is taken to determine the bilirubin count. According to Dr. Erlichman, the skin color is affected once the bilirubin level reaches 9. If the bilirubin count remains below 15, he says, the condition will probably resolve itself.

Many doctors feel that if the bilirubin count is under 15 and going down, the bris may be performed. According to Rabbi Yosef David Weisberg, national supervisor of Israel's governmental commission in charge of *mohalim*, the custom in Jerusalem is to perform the bris if the bilirubin count is 12 or under and on the way down.[19]

Sometimes the yellowness can be a sign of a different illness, in which case the bris may be performed only seven days after the baby has recovered.[20]

If the newborn was in need of a blood transfusion, the bris may not be performed until seven days have passed after recovery.[21]

A bilirubin level higher than 15 requires medical intervention in the form of phototherapy. The infant is placed in a special bassinet and exposed to various wavelengths of light to decompose bilirubin in the skin. Phototherapy is usually successful in bringing down the bilirubin count within one or two days. During this time the baby can continue to nurse as usual. However, in the case of breast-feeding-related jaundice, which occurs on day 5 or 6 after birth, a 24- to 48-hour cessation from breast feeding is required. In cases where the infant is treated for jaundice, the newborn is considered sick and requires the seven-day waiting period after he ceases the phototherapy.[22]

For individual cases, parents should consult their pediatrician and their Rav.

The Covenant "And God said to Avraham: You shall keep My Covenant, you and your seed after you, throughout their generations."[23] Avraham *Avinu* was commanded to enter the Covenant with God, symbolizing an unbreakable bond connecting Avraham and his descendants with Hashem. From that moment on there would be a People that would bear the stamp of Hashem on their flesh. They would be chosen to teach monotheism and ethics to the entire world. The bris is an everlasting statement that the bearer is one of God's Chosen.

The bris is performed upon the reproductive organ to symbolize that this attribute is inherent.[24] Every child born to a Jewish mother possesses it, and at eight days after birth, every Jewish male child enters the Covenant by having the sign of the bris made on his flesh. As God told Avraham: "And he that is eight days old shall be circumcised among you, every male throughout your generations."[25]

Despite the decrees of Antiochus outlawing *bris milah*, and throughout the expulsions and persecutions that our Nation suffered in exile, the Jewish People never ceased to perform this mitzvah. To this day, virtually all Jews, regardless of their level of religious commitment, observe this beloved commandment with zealousness and joy, thereby fulfilling the words of *Chazal*: "Every mitzvah for which the Jews were willing to make the supreme sacrifice, such as *bris milah*, will always be observed by them"; and: "Every mitzvah that the Jews accepted with joy, such as *bris milah*, will always be fulfilled with joy."[26]

NOTES

1. R. Yitzchak Lipietz, *Sefer Matamim.*
2. *Berachos* 13a.
3. Talmud Yerushalmi, ch. 4, *halachah* 3, *Sukkah* 4:3.
4. *Devarim* 6:4.
5. *Pesachim* 56a.
6. Rashi, *Bereshis* 46:29.
7. *Berachos* 61b.
8. This story was told to Rabbi Finkelstein personally by the soldier himself as they lay side-by-side in the hospital.
9. *Sifsei Chachamim, Berachos* 13a.

10. Netziv, *Amek Ha-Davar, Bereshis* 46:29. And this is why Ya'akov said the Shema when he saw his son Yosef after all those years — in order to prepare himself for the reunion and enable him to bow down to the viceroy of Egypt: his son.

11. This custom is called *Bris Yitzchak.*

12. Rama, *Yoreh De'ah* 265:12.

13. Taz, *Yoreh De'ah* 265:13.

14. *Yoreh De'ah* 262:2.

15. *Iggros Moshe, Yoreh De'ah*, vol. II, 121. However, if he was put into an incubator for a short time after birth in order to warm him up, he is not considered sick (Dr. Avraham Steinberg, *Encyclopedia of Jewish Medical Ethics*, vol. III, p. 694).

16. Heard from Dr. Matityahu Erlichman; see *Tzitz Eliezer*, vol. XIII, 82, which says in the name of Dr. Avraham that a fever of 99.5°F (37.5°C) (and even less than that) is considered high fever.

17. See *Iggros Moshe, Yoreh De'ah*, vol. II, 121; see also *Tzitz Eliezer*, vol. XIII, 82.

18. *Yoreh De'ah* 263:1.

19. Heard from Rabbi Weisberg in the name of Rabbi Y.S. Elyashiv, and from Rabbi S.Z. Auerbach.

20. *Tzitz Eliezer*, vol. XIII, 81; and heard from Dr. Erlichman.

21. *Iggros Moshe, Yoreh De'ah*, vol. II, 121.

22. For according to Dr. Erlichman, at this point the baby is considered healthy. It is very likely that the custom regarding this particular problem will change as medical research into jaundice develops. Even today there are different opinions. For further information, see Dr. Avraham Steinberg, *Encyclopedia of Jewish Medical Ethics*, vol. III, p. 698.

23. *Bereshis* 17:9.

24. *Sefer Ha-Chinnuch*, mitzvah 2.

25. *Bereshis* 17:12.

26. *Shabbos* 130a.

21 | It's a Girl!

Far beyond pearls is her value.
MISHLEI 31:10

Although there is no set time for celebrating the birth of a baby girl, it is appropriate to make a *simchah* when a family is blessed with a daughter.[1] In fact, the arrival of a daughter is an immediate *simchah* in itself.

Many people wonder why Jewish girls do not carry a sign of the Covenant on their bodies as men do. After all, since circumcision is such an important aspect of Judaism, why shouldn't a woman — who is just as much a part of *Am Yisrael* as a man is — have an everlasting *os* ("sign") on her body as well?

Born "Circumcised"

Chazal explain that a Jewish woman is born as if she were (already) circumcised,[2] that is, free of impurity.

The foreskin (*orlah*) is a symbol of impurity, and must therefore be cut off. Until the foreskin is detached, the body is considered incomplete. That is why we do not name the child until after the bris: so that his name will not be "attached" to his impurity.

Clearly, if Hashem had so desired, He could have created man already circumcised — already "completed," but He wanted man to play an active role in his own creation. Hashem wanted *us* to complete our bodies, an action symbolizing our constant efforts to perfect our souls. Although we were born with a soul that has the capacity to be "Godly," it requires tireless toil in order to fulfill that potential.[3] In that sense, our soul, like our body, is incomplete, and we must likewise "circumcise" our soul to remove impurity.

The Talmud's assertion that a woman is considered circumcised means that she possesses a soul that is more perfect than that of a man, a soul that by nature is closer to Godliness. The "shell" of impurity does not cover the woman as it does her male counterpart, so she needs no circumcision.

On the verse: "And Moshe went up unto God and the Lord called out of the mountain, saying: 'This shall you say to the House of Ya'akov and tell to the Children of Yisrael'"[4] Chazal comment that "the House of Ya'akov" (Beis Ya'akov) are the women.[5] Note the use of the softer expression, "say to," in conjunction with Beis Ya'akov, as opposed to the harsher expression, "tell to," which is used in conjunction with Bnei Yisrael. This implies that Moshe was commanded to speak more softly to the women. The Maharal makes the following observation: Beis Ya'akov was addressed before the men because their guarantee of reward is greater than that of the men. That is also the reason that Moshe was told to speak gently to the women, for their reward is earned in a gentler, more natural fashion. To the men, however, he had to speak harshly, alluding to the hard life of constant Torah study — day and night — they would have to endure in order to earn their reward.[6]

Both men and women are required to yearn for the fulfillment of sitting in the House of the Lord all the days of their life — in this world and in the next. A man's "House of the Lord" is the beis midrash, the house of Torah study. A woman's "House of the Lord" can be her own home, as it is written: "She anticipates the ways of her household."[7] In order to achieve this she must imbue her family with the spirit of Torah and the warmth of chesed (kindness). She must generate enthusiasm in her family members for fulfilling mitzvos, and the loving anticipation of the *Yamim Tovim.*

Just like Hashem, Who is *Koneh Ha-Kol* ("creates everything") and *Gomel Chasadim Tovim* ("bestows beneficial kindness"),[8] a woman brings new life into the world from the inner chambers of her body. Her offspring are then raised with an innate desire to bestow kindness. Since the very essence of a woman is to give, she requires no circumcision.

Another reason that a woman does not need an *os* on her body is because Hashem intended that man and woman should marry and become one flesh. Thus, a woman is connected to the bris of her husband. **Man and Woman: One Flesh** Man and woman form a union, each one compensating for the shortcomings of the other. Without his wife, the full significance of the man's bris is limited. The presence of the sign of the Covenant on man's reproductive organ symbolizes the inherent nature of the "chosenness" of the Jewish People, but that is obtained only if his wife is Jewish. The "chosenness" of the Jewish People is passed on through the Jewish mother only. It is the mother who transmits the Jewish soul; the father makes the Covenant.

Having a baby girl is therefore an occasion for immediate happiness: She is born with the spiritual potential that needs no circumcision, and right away she is given a name, to be counted among *Am Yisrael.* (See Chapter 22 on Naming Your Child.)

The love of a father for his daughter is very great. To a father, every daughter is a treasure, a jewel. **Father and Daughter** Even if he wanted a son, once his daughter has arrived it won't be long before a very special relationship is established between them. From that point on, he is won over. The Gemara says that a father loses sleep worrying about his daughter. He worries about her safety and happiness.[9] *Chazal* say that a person only worries about someone or something that is very important in his life

— only someone that he loves and cares for very much. This worrying never stops; it lasts his whole life long.[10] It seems that a daughter always remains "Daddy's little girl."

A Treasure Needs Protection   A daughter's safety and happiness are a constant major concern for parents. It affects the way they run their household and even their bank accounts. Since little girls are so vulnerable to physical and emotional harm, parents tend to be more protective of their daughters than of their sons. *Chazal* recognize this factor and interpret the Priestly Blessing in the following manner: "May God bless you and protect you" — "bless you" means you should have sons, and "protect you" means you should have daughters, because daughters require protection.[11] Does this mean that sons are not in need of protection, or that daughters are not a blessing? Surely not. What it means is that the emphasis is placed on that which is most lacking. Daughters are *already* a *berachah*, as the Talmud says: Every *berachah* in a man's house is because of his wife.[12] The ability to imbue a home with *berachah* is a Jewish woman's birthright. But because of her vulnerability to physical and emotional harm, she needs protection. Sons are less vulnerable, so they do not require the emphasis of protection, but they do require blessing.

The Most Beautiful Maidaleh   The birth of a daughter is a great *simchah*. She will, with Hashem's help, grow to become one of the pillars that support the world, a part of the foundation of the whole Jewish Nation, as she will build her own household with ethical Torah values.

But right now, to her parents she will simply be a bundle of joy, a priceless treasure. She will charm you with her smiles and warm you with her affection. She will turn your house into a kindergarten, and she will enchant you with her eagerness to do mitzvos. She will break your heart when she feels hurt and she will gladden you when she is happy. She will look so lovely in her new Shabbos dress and she will always be the most beautiful *maidaleh* in the world. She will always be there to help, and she will be faithful through your old age.

Mazal tov on your new jewel.

NOTES

1. *Sefer Matamim; see* Hebrew appendix.
2. *Avodah Zarah* 27a.
3. *Sefer Ha-Chinnuch,* mitzvah 2.
4. *Shemos* 19:3.
5. *Midrash Rabbah* on this verse.
6. Maharal, exposition on the Torah (*Mahaduras Yerushalayim* 27).
7. *Mishlei* 31:27; *see* the commentary of the Vilna Gaon.
8. The *Shemoneh Esreh* prayer.
9. *Sanhedrin* 100b.
10. Ibid.
11. *Bemidbar Rabbah* 11:5.
12. *Bava Metzia* 59a.

22 | Naming Your Child

*One should always be careful to choose a
name for his child suitable to the child's
potential righteousness...the name can
have either a good or bad influence.*

MIDRASH TANCHUMA, PARASHAS HA'AZINU

New parents want to choose a name for their child which
is both meaningful and appealing. The Torah attaches
great significance to a name, and teaches that it is important to give a name which will have a good influence.

A name can be chosen at the parents' descretion. Although there are no set rules, there are customs that
may help you. You can give a Biblical name, or a Hebrew
name derived from nature, or a name in memory of someone. But you should never use a *rasha*'s name, no matter how nice it is.[1] Some authorities forbid non-Jewish
names,[2] while others allow translations (Ya'akov-Jacob).[3]

It is the Ashkenazi custom to name the baby in memory of one's deceased parents and/or grandparents, with
the hope that all their good attributes will be carried on
in the infant. Another reason is that naming a child after
the deceased can have a positive effect (*ilui neshamah*)
on the soul of the departed.[4] The Sephardic custom is to
honor the grandparents even during their lifetimes, by
giving the baby his grandparent's name.

It is also customary to name children after one's
teachers and rabbis.[5] One should consult a Rav about
naming a child in memory of a person who died young.[6]

Some choose a name from the Torah portion of the

week in which the child was born, or from a Festival that falls on or near the date: Mordechai for a boy born on Purim, Ruth for a girl born on Shavuos, or Menachem/Nechamah for a child born on Tisha B'Av.

Choosing a name should not be the cause of a quarrel. If the parents do not agree, there are customs they can follow. A common Ashkenazic custom is that the mother chooses a name for the first child, the father for the second, and so forth, alternating with each birth. If you are in doubt as to your family's or community's custom, consult a Rav. The overriding consideration should be *shalom bayis*.[7]

It is most important not to give your child a name that may be a source of ridicule as he grows up. No matter whom you would like to name him after, and no matter how beautiful or meaningful the name may appear to you, you are not doing your child a kindness if you give him a name that will cause him humiliation and anguish. Parents who like off-beat and obscure names should think hard about their choice.

The Influence of a Name

One cannot help but note the emphasis given to names in the Torah. It provides us with long lists of names,[8] and sometimes goes out of its way to give us an explanation for the name. For example: "And Leah conceived, and bore a son and she called his name *Re'uven*, for she said, '*Ki ra'ah Hashem b'onyi* — Surely Hashem has seen my affliction'" (*Bereshis* 29:32).

Sometimes a name can affect the child's character, and his future. We see this in *Megillas Ruth*, where the Hebrew roots of "Machlon" and "Kilyon" foreshadow their tragic death: "Machlon was *erased* from the world, and Kilyon was *destroyed*." Naomi's name suggests her fine character: "Naomi, for her deeds were *na'im u-ne'imim* (nice and pleasant)."[9]

A Name Divinely Given

When Avraham *Avinu* was told he would have a son, he was also told what to name him: "You should call him Yitzchak" (*Bereshis* 17:19). Because of the extreme importance of a name,

Hashem Himself wanted to name the first baby born to enter the Covenant with God at eight days of age.[10]

After Yitzchak, everyone was allowed to name his own child. Even so, we do not really choose the name ourselves, for Hashem is a partner in naming every child. The Ari z"l said, "None of the names in the world are coincidental." Those who think that children receive names at random are mistaken. Hashem must approve of every name, and that name then becomes associated with the character or actions of the person.[11] For this reason, selecting a name requires careful consideration.

It is customary to name a boy at his *bris milah*. Various customs apply to naming a girl. The most common is to name her at the first Torah-reading after the birth or on the first Shabbos.[12]

Every Star a Name   David *Ha-Melech* wrote in *Tehillim* (147:4): "He counts the number of the stars; He gives a name to each of them." Since the beginning of time, the stars have captured mankind's imagination. They hold the secrets of creation, and of the future. They are a road map to the navigator, a challenge to the astronomer, and a symbol of quest to the explorer.

Those sparkling lights in the vast darkness seem so small, yet we know they are not. Their numbers reach infinity, but all are special to Hashem, and He gives each a name. Each has its unique purpose, and no two are exactly the same.

The Torah often compares the Jewish People to the stars (*Bereshis* 15:5). For just as the stars illuminate the darkness of night, so the Jewish People enlighten the darkness of the world with the truth of Torah. Just as stars guide travelers along their way, the Jewish People give moral and ethical direction to mankind.

As the stars hold the secrets of the future, world history revolves around the Jewish People, leading inexorably to the final Redemption. Just as massive stars appear tiny, so the Jewish People seem insignificant in comparison to a world population of billions. Yet there

exists an underlying understanding of the contributing
force and massive potential of *Am Yisrael.*

Hashem gives names to each star for they are dear to
Him, and likewise He takes part in naming every Jew.
Like the stars, no two Jewish souls are exactly alike.
Every Jew has his unique function and special mitzvah
in which he excels. Every Jew shines a different light.

In the days of Redemption, the love of Hashem for His
children will be ever so clear. As we read in the *haftarah*
after every Tisha B'Av on *Shabbos Nachamu:* "Lift up
your eyes on high and behold Who has created these
things [the stars], that bring out their host by number.
He calls them all by names; because of the greatness of
His might and because He is strong in power, not one is
missing" (*Yeshayahu* 40:26).

At the final Redemption, every Jew will return to Jerusalem — not one will be missing. Each one will again
be counted, and to each one *Hashem will give a name.*

NOTES

1. *Yoma* 38b; Rabbi Yosef David Weisberg, *Otzar Ha-Bris,* "*Zeh
   shemi l'olam*" 5:1.
2. *Darchei Teshuvah* 178:14.
3. *Responsa, Tzofnas Pane'ach* 275, cited in *Otzar Ha-Bris* 6:1.
4. *Responsa, Ein Yehudah* 12, cited in *Otzar Ha-Bris* 4:1.
5. *See Otzar Ha-Bris,* pp. 208-20.
6. *Iggros Moshe, Yoreh De'ah,* vol. II, 122.
7. *Ateres Shalom,* pp. 25, 27.
8. *Bereshis* 29:32.
9. *Ruth Rabbah* 20; *see also Maggid Mesharim, Parashas Shemos.*
10. *See* Rashi, *Bereshis* 25:26; Hashem also gave Ya'akov his name.
11. *Amud Shamayim* 4, cited in *Otzar Ha-Bris,* p. 207; *see* R. Yis-
    rael Hess, *Derech Emunah,* p. 15.
12. *See Responsa, Tzitz Eliezer,* vol. XIII, 20; *see also Responsa,
    Minchas Yitzchak,* vol. IV, 107; *see* Hebrew appendix.

23 | Feeding Your Baby

What constitutes a baby's nourishment during his first years? His mother's milk, milk that is his without effort, without preparation. Similarly, the manna nourished the Jewish People during their first years of nationhood in the desert: 'Behold I will rain bread from heaven for you...and it was like the coriander seed, white, and the taste of it was like wafers made with honey.'

R. BETZALEL NAOR, YECHIDAH SHE'B'NEFESH

During pregnancy you provide nourishment for your baby passively and automatically. Once your baby is born, however, you will have to take a more active role in providing for his nutritional needs. Of course, you will want to give your newborn the best, most suitable form of nutrition.

It is common knowledge that breast feeding is considered the finest source of nourishment for an infant. Although nursing can be time-consuming and at times physically draining, the enormous benefits both for you and for your baby surely outweigh the relatively minor difficulties that may come your way.

Benefits for Baby Breast milk is specifically suited to your baby's digestive needs. Its lower, yet adequate, protein level can be readily absorbed and utilized by a baby's body, whereas the extra protein in cow's milk must be processed in his body and excreted. In addition, the soft curds formed by breast milk facilitate digestion and prevent constipation.[1]

Nursing prevents illness in babies, and helps to promote recovery when illness does occur. Protective antibodies and anti-viral properties are passed from mother to baby through breast milk. The newborn thus gains a passive immunity against many infectious diseases, filling the void until his own immune system becomes fully functional at 3-4 months.[2] The immunological properties of breast milk (IgA antibodies) also help prevent digestive tract infections during the first 6-12 months of life, and aid in the process of recovery from illness.[3] Moreover, breast feeding supplies a natural protection against milk allergies, which are common in formula-fed infants. Nursing even appears to reduce the risk of certain chronic diseases. It has been proven beneficial to both the premature and full-term newborn.[4]

Breast feeding encourages optimal mouth and jaw development while exercising cheek muscles, mouth and tongue.[5] This exertion helps to prepare the tongue and mouth for proper speech. It also aids in the prevention of "tongue thrust," an abnormal swallowing pattern common among bottle-fed infants due to the pressure of the baby's tongue against the nipple of the bottle to prevent choking from too strong a flow. Thus problems associated with "tongue thrust" — such as mouth-breathing, lip-biting, gum disease and orthodontic problems — are usually avoided in the breast-fed baby.

Breast milk is the ultimate health food.[6] It flows from the breast practically germ-free, containing no synthetic components, preservatives, or artificial ingredients.

A breast-fed baby cannot be overfed because mother's milk is the perfect food with the most suitable caloric value for your baby. *Chazal* say, "Breast milk is the primary source of nourishment, and anything else is secondary. Similarly, the manna was the primary nourishment of the Children of Israel in the desert. Even if a baby nurses all day long, it will not be harmed, and will even derive benefit from it. The same was true of the manna — even if *Am Yisrael* ate it all day long, they were not harmed by it."[7]

Benefits for Mother Breast milk is always ready, conveniently at the right temperature, and free, as opposed to the complicated routine necessary to prepare high-priced infant formulas in bottles.

During the nursing experience, there is a constant flow of love between mother and baby. The physical benefits for the mother are numerous. The tactile stimulation and cuddling involved in nursing enhance mother-baby bonding. The connection is so strong that even a blind baby recognizes his own mother by taste and smell.[8] In addition, baby's sucking stimulates the uterus to contract and accelerates its return to pre-pregnancy size (uterine involution).

Studies conducted by the American Cancer Society show that the incidence of breast cancer is lower in women who have breast-fed their infants. Furthermore, although breast feeding is not a reliable form of birth control, ovulation (and menstruation) can be suspended for many months, even up to a year or more.

Breast Feeding: How It Works The breast is composed of mammary glands which in turn consist of alveoli and secreting cells that produce milk. The milk produced in the alveolar cells flows to reservoirs located behind the nipple. Milk issues forth from fifteen to twenty tiny openings in the nipple.

The nipple is surrounded by a circle called the areola. During pregnancy the glands in the areola (Montgomery's glands) become enlarged and secrete a substance which lubricates and protects the nipple while nursing. Once breast feeding stops, the glands recede, and the nipple and areola lighten to about one shade darker than their original pre-pregnancy color.

When the placenta is delivered, the estrogen and progesterone levels in the body drop sharply. This drop signals the pituitary gland to release the hormone pro-lactin, which causes the mammary glands to produce milk.

Baby's sucking stimulates the pituitary glands to continue to release prolactin and another hormone, oxyto-cin. While prolactin makes the milk, oxytocin causes the alveoli cells to contract, squeezing the milk into the reservoirs behind the nipple and making it available to the baby.

The passage of milk into these reservoirs is known as the "let-down" reflex. As the baby begins to suck, the mother will feel the let-down reflex, which is commonly accompanied by a tingling, tugging sensation of the breast.

The let-down reflex may be stimulated even before the mother begins to nurse her baby, when, for example, she hears his cry or thinks of him. When this happens, the milk may drip freely from the breast, wetting through the mother's clothes. Nursing pads offer some protection for clothing until the mother's body becomes accustomed to a nursing routine. Then such accidents will occur less frequently. The sensation of the let-down reflex usually diminishes after the first few months of nursing. In problem cases, it is possible to stimulate a slow let-down reflex with the use of an oxytocin nasal spray.

Colostrum

From the 16th week of pregnancy, a thin, yellowish fluid can be expressed from the breasts. This antecedent of milk production is known as colostrum. It is composed of protein, sugar, fat, water, minerals, and vitamins, and is rich in maternal antibodies. Its low sugar and fat content make it the ideal food for the first few days of life. Colostrum is nutritionally balanced to enable the newborn's delicate digestive system to function and even to pass meconium from his bowel.[9]

You need not worry that there is nothing in your breasts to feed your baby after delivery. A supplemental bottle is totally unnecessary. Colostrum fulfills your newborn's total nutritional needs during those first few days, and is replaced by true milk within 24-72 hours after delivery. The sooner and more frequently you nurse, the sooner the milk will come in.

Preparation for Lactation You are most likely reading this book during the nine months of waiting to give birth. It may seem hard to imagine that it will finally be over and that you will, God willing, have the responsibility of feeding a newborn. Pregnancy, however, is the time to start preparing yourself physically and psychologically for nursing your baby.

PHYSICAL PREPARATION

To physically prepare the breasts you should wear a supportive and properly fitted bra throughout the pregnancy and lactation period. During the month before your due date, strengthen and moisturize your nipples once a day by applying a fingertip of lanolin ointment or Vitamin E oil to the nipples and gently rolling and pulling them outward, imitating what the baby will do when he nurses. This can be especially helpful for women with flat or inverted nipples.

PSYCHOLOGICAL PREPARATION

Psychological preparation for nursing is just as important as physical preparation. Even during the early stages of pregnancy, a woman should understand the importance of nursing. Talking to other nursing mothers can be very helpful. A positive psychological perception will enable you to overcome any difficulties which may arise, and ensure a successful nursing relationship with your baby. This relationship is so important that the *kohanim* in the time of the *Beis Hamikdash* would pray for lactating mothers to be successful in their nursing.[10] With a positive attitude, you too will be successful!

Beginning Breast Feeding It is usually recommended to nurse the newborn immediately after birth. If your baby's color, respiration and temperature are normal, and you are feeling well, then you should be allowed to breast feed on the delivery bed.

You don't have to sit up. Just turn on your side, cuddle the baby in the crook of your arm and brush your baby's cheek with your finger or breast. When baby's cheek is touched, his "rooting" reflex will be stimulated, and he will search for the breast. Gently glide the nipple with forefinger and thumb into baby's mouth. Make sure that he engulfs the entire nipple and areola, causing his mouth to appear to be open. If he is latching on properly, you should feel a pulling sensation on the nipple.

The baby should then begin to suck. If his nose is covered, you may need to use your first two fingers to depress the top of the breast away from his nose, allowing him to breathe comfortably.

Every newborn is different. Some are hungry, some disinterested, and others sleepy from medication. Although this initial nursing and bonding experience is a nice way to get acquainted, if your baby seems disinterested or you are not feeling up to nursing, you can postpone this first feeding. The main thing is to be relaxed and enjoy getting to know one another.

To release the baby's mouth from the nipple, insert your pinky in his mouth and pull the breast toward you. This will let your baby know to release the suction and will prevent any injury to the nipple by abruptly pulling the baby off the breast.

After a cesarean section, a mother can also nurse as soon as she feels up to it. With a little assistance and pillows to get comfortable, a post-cesarean mother's nursing experience will be as successful as any other mother's.

Ask the nursery nurses to refrain from giving bottles. Placing a small sign in the bassinet is an effective way to communicate this request. Don't be afraid that your nursing success will be spoiled by nighttime bottles or by the initial bottle of water he may receive after delivery. As annoying as some hospital routines can be, remember that it's only for two or three days.

Some hospitals offer the "rooming-in" option. You and

your baby will be hospitalized together in the same room, allowing you to nurse on demand and care for your baby to your mutual satisfaction.

Of course, once you are home, everything literally "flows" much more smoothly, as it is easier to relax in your own home.

At your convenience, you may experiment with a number of positions for nursing besides sitting up: lying on your stomach, on your side, or on your back. Make yourself more comfortable by supporting yourself with pillows. When nursing while in a sitting position, do not slump forward onto your baby. Use pillows and/or the arms of the chair to bring the baby to breast-level. This will prevent fatigue and muscle strain.

To keep the milk supply evenly distributed, nurse on one breast for 5-10 minutes and then switch to the other. Every day increase the amount of time your baby nurses at each breast. When he is finished nursing, the second breast will remain slightly fuller than the first breast, so remember to begin the next feeding with the side on which you finished nursing the previous time. You may want to place a safety pin on your bra strap to remind you.

The hospital's routine of feeding every 3-4 hours often falls by the wayside once mother and baby arrive home. It is not uncommon for a newborn to want to nurse as often as every 2 hours.

Breast Care   After delivery, avoid using any creams or lotions, including lanolin, on the nipples. It is soothing to apply a drop of Vitamin E oil after each feeding, and this need not be wiped away before nursing. If you want to clean the breasts before and after a feeding, use lukewarm water and wipe the nipples gently with a clean cloth or gauze. Avoid using soap on the breasts.

Possible Difficulties   Although breast feeding has been the natural and acceptable way to feed newborns since the beginning of time, there are difficulties that may crop up. Fortunately, these can be easily overcome.

ENGORGEMENT

Engorgement is a fairly common occurrence from the third to fifth day after delivery. The breasts become hot, heavy, full and hard because of the increased blood and lymph supply, not due to an overabundance of milk. Although engorgement is not caused by too much milk, draining milk from the breasts either manually or by frequent nursing is the treatment of choice.

Sometimes the breast becomes so hard that it is difficult for the baby to attach himself. To soften the breast, take a hot shower or apply wet, warm washcloths half an hour before nursing. Place one hand beneath and one hand on top of the breast, and gently massage using a forward motion, until some milk is expressed and the fullness subsides. Now it will be easier for the baby to grasp the nipple, and the breast will be softer to the touch. You will be able to nurse with less discomfort to you and baby.

If your breasts still feel full after nursing, manually express milk until you feel relief from the fullness. Engorgement should subside in 24-48 hours.

SORE NIPPLES

During the first or second week, when the new mother is just beginning to nurse, sore nipples are a common problem. Fair-haired and light-complected women are most prone to develop sore nipples. The strongest discomfort is felt when the baby first latches on, but it subsides with the continuation of the nursing session.

In order to prevent increased soreness and possible fissures (cracks) in the nipples, here are some helpful suggestions:

❧ Check that the baby has taken the nipple and most of the areola into his mouth and is not just chewing on the nipple.

❧ Do not leave the nipples wet and soggy. Change

nursing pads and bras frequently, and do not use nursing pads or bras with plastic linings.

❦ Try to expose the nipples to air between feedings or wear a loose-fitting garment without a bra.

❦ Take two acetaminophen (Tylenol/Acamol) tablets before each feeding to relieve discomfort.

❦ Express a bit of milk immediately before the baby establishes contact, so that he will not have to suck so hard.

❦ Nurse the less sore side first and limit nursing to five minutes on the sore side.

Do not stop nursing. If a scab develops, don't pick at it. Contact a breast-feeding counselor through your hospital or local La Leche League for assistance at the first sign of difficulty.

MASTITIS

Breast infections can occur at any time during a mother's nursing career, but usually do not appear before the third or fourth week after delivery. A clogged milk duct or staphylococcal infection which originates from the baby and is transmitted to the mother are the most common causes of infection.

The indications of mastitis are: flu-like symptoms, fever, and the affected breast becoming hot, red and tender. Pain can even radiate to the underarm area.

The treatment of choice is bed rest, an increase in fluid intake and *continuing to nurse.*[11] Rest is crucial to recovery and also provides the perfect opportunity to nurse frequently. You need not fear that the baby will become ill if you nurse while you have an infection as he naturally harbors this same germ. Nursing will actually relieve some of the symptoms and keep your milk flowing. A hot compress is also soothing.

You can take acetaminophen (Tylenol/Acamol) for fever reduction and pain relief, but check with your doctor (family physician or obstetrician) to see if he recommends antibiotics for the infection.

A breast abscess is an uncommon complication of mastitis which may require a temporary cessation of nursing from the affected breast. Medical care and antibiotics are necessary.

The nursing infant drinks up to half a quart of breast milk per day. When speaking of such a quantity, it is easy to visualize that drugs which pass into the breast milk can have significant effects on a baby.[12] In a study of 400 mothers who drank liquor, it was found that enough alcohol was consumed by their babies through the breast milk to impede the infants' motor development, slowing progress in learning to crawl and walk. Whether these effects are temporary or permanent is still unknown.[13]

Medication while Nursing

Although there are some drugs which will not detrimentally affect the baby, it is important for all nursing mothers to consult a pediatrician before taking any over-the-counter or prescription drugs.

Successful breast feeding is not dependent on breast size or physical characteristics. If you are physically and psychologically prepared to breast feed, you will have milk. It is indeed extremely rare for a postpartum woman not to have milk. A woman's milk supply is diminished when she is tired, nervous, worried or simply doesn't want to nurse.

Milk Supply

The Gemara tells us that whoever can give birth can nurse.[14] Channah used this information to her advantage in her prayer to Hashem: "Everything You created has a purpose...breasts to nurse. My breasts that were put near my heart, what purpose have they? Give me a child, and I will nurse with them" (*Berachos* 31b).

According to an article in the *American Journal of Disease in Children*, the most common reason for weaning at any age is a perceived lack of breast milk.[15] It must be understood, therefore, that the quantity of breast milk is based on a supply-and-demand system. The amount of milk produced by the breasts increases according to how frequently you nurse, resulting in a greater ability to supply your baby's nutritional needs. This is important to remember if you want to maintain your milk supply or increase the amount of milk you have to offer your baby. Even in the heat of the summer, you are capable of providing all the fluid your infant needs just by continuing to nurse.

The Radak, in his commentary on *Tehillim* (8:3), says that Hashem's supervision is evident even in the smallest aspect of existence. A tiny baby enters the world and instantly we can witness wonders: his mother is able to nurse him, and the flow of milk is regulated according to his needs, capacity and ability to suckle.

Some mothers are concerned that their babies are not getting enough milk. You can be sure that your baby is getting what he needs if he is producing at least five wet diapers a day, seems content, and gains weight at a steady pace.

Even if weight gain does not keep up with the clinical graph, an infant who progresses developmentally is also meeting his nutritional requirements. Supplementation for an infant who is truly underweight depends upon the age of the baby. Formula or solid foods may be instituted into the diet. A doctor or pediatric nurse should be consulted.

Nutrition and the Nursing Mother

Following a judicious nutritional routine during pregnancy and nursing will improve the quality of your milk.[16] The Gemara in *Kesubbos* (60b) encourages the nursing mother to eat more for her own sake and for the sake of the baby. Rashi adds that a woman who eats more will produce more milk.

In order to support the delicate supply-and-demand system, you must make sure that your diet includes enough fluids and good food. You need approximately 25% more of the same nutrients and fluids you so carefully consumed during pregnancy. A daily increase of 500 calories is recommended to sustain breast feeding.[17] Research indicates that although fluid intake may not directly affect the volume of breast milk, a woman's body will supply milk even at the expense of dehydrating its own tissues. A good way to get enough to drink is to have a glass of water, milk or juice before or during each nursing session.

As in pregnancy, the lactation period is not the time to go on a diet to lose weight. You must eat sensibly in order to maintain your milk supply. Through proper eating, however, the weight gained in pregnancy will gradually burn off, especially as you are busy nursing and caring for your newborn.

The baby is directly affected by the quality and type of food you eat. The Talmud relates that while the Children of Israel were in the desert, the manna would taste like any food at all, except foods that were bad for nursing mothers.[18]

The Gemara in *Kesubbos* (60b) specifically advises against eating foods which are bad for the milk. Since we do not know to which foods the Gemara is referring, anything which may potentially cause your infant stomach upset or allergies should be avoided. If you notice an increase in the baby's fussiness, analyze what you have recently eaten. You might want to avoid those foods in the future.

In addition to affecting your baby physically, the foods you eat also have a spiritual effect. The Rama writes that if a woman eats non-kosher food — even if she is allowed to for medical purposes — she should not nurse immediately afterwards. This is because the non-kosher food can engender negative characteristics in the human being.[19]

If you feel that your milk supply is dwindling and that you yourself are depleted, perhaps this is due not just to a lack of proper and sufficient food and fluid, but also to a lack of rest. Although not easily accomplished with a new baby in the house, getting adequate rest is a basic requirement for successful nursing. During the initial few months, in addition to the de-

Rest and Energy

mands of nursing, your body is still recuperating from pregnancy and childbirth.

Just as you exert the energy to prepare meals for your family, your body is constantly exerting itself to provide an adequate milk supply for your baby. You must restore this energy through eating properly and getting enough rest.

Pumping and Storage   Even if you go to work or miss a feeding or two for whatever reason, you can still provide your baby with a bottle of your own breast milk. Breast milk can be expressed in three ways: manually, with a hand pump, or with an electric pump.

Manually expressing milk is not complicated but requires a bit of practice. To learn this art, it is worthwhile to seek advice from an experienced mother or a breast-feeding counselor.

A hand pump is inexpensive and can be bought in any pharmacy. Easy-to-follow instructions are provided in order to guide you. Electric pumps are used in hospitals and can also be rented for home use. Suction strength may be adjusted, but it frequently takes a few trial runs until you become accustomed to its action. It is important to wash your hands before starting any milk expression and to keep all equipment absolutely clean.

Expressed milk can be stored for future use or donated to a milk bank (for sick or premature infants who need breast milk). Use a sterile plastic bottle, or better yet, the disposable plastic liners made for some brands of baby bottles. To sterilize, place the bottles in boiling water for 15 minutes, nipples for 5 minutes. Alternatively, both can be sterilized in the dishwasher by going through one complete cycle.

Breast milk can be refrigerated for up to 24 hours or stored frozen in a refrigerator freezer for two weeks. Milk can also be stored in a deep-freeze for up to two years.

Nursing a baby is a beautiful way to express one's **Tzenius** femininity. The Gemara says that David *Ha-Melech* **(Modesty)** would look at his mother's breasts while nursing **when Nursing** and say *Shirah.*[20] The *Midrash* explains that in animals it is natural to suckle from a point near the womb, but a woman's breasts are set off in a beautiful and more respectable place, so that her baby nurses from a place of honor.[21]

When you are at home, all you need to do to respond to your baby's nursing needs is simply to find a comfortable place to nurse. But what about when you are away from home or in someone else's home? The Talmud tells us that Rabbi Meir spoke very strongly against women who nursed in public.[22] No matter where a nursing mother finds herself, she must nurse in a modest and discreet fashion, and not expose herself unnecessarily.

In some situations, however, it may be unavoidable to nurse in public; the baby may not be able to wait for a more appropriate setting. In these cases, one must exercise careful judgment. A good provision is to always carry a light receiving blanket or towel with which to cover yourself.

When nursing in your husband's presence (which **Tzenius at** is permissible if you are not a *niddah*), he is forbid- **Home** den to say *Keri'as Shema* or other sacred words.[23] However, he may close his eyes or turn away to say them.[24] A nursing mother may recite sacred words while nursing[25] (providing she did not touch the normally covered parts of her body).

There is no argument that "breast is best," but **The Bottle-** there are a number of reasons why a mother will **Feeding** choose to feed her baby with formula. Even if a **Option** woman chooses to bottle feed one child, she may decide to nurse her next one. As we discussed earlier, breast feeding requires a good deal of psychological preparation. A new mother may be overwhelmed with caring for a newborn or may feel she needs to give her time and attention to older children. Work, ill health, or chronic medications may also prevent a woman from breast feeding.

Peer pressure to nurse can be a very persuasive factor, but a woman should not allow herself to be judged by others. She needs to decide what is best for herself and her baby. Giving a baby a bottle enables a mother — or any family member — to cuddle and be close.

According to pediatrician Dr. M. Erlichman, baby formula is a good substitute for breast milk. It is strongly recommended to avoid giving regular cow's milk before 6 months, and preferably not until 9 months. There are even some doctors who maintain that bottle-fed babies should remain on formula until their first birthday.

One should make sure that the formula has added vitamins and iron so supplementation is not necessary. Nursing infants may need iron supplements at about 9 months, pending the results of a routine blood test of hemoglobin at age 6-7 months.

Formula Requirements   Formula requirements are easy to assess. First, you need to know how much your baby weighs.

Of course, there may be one meal when your baby will eat more or less than his "allotted" amount. Be flexible. Just as we adults have more of an appetite at certain meals and less at other meals, the same is true of infants.

U.S. MEASURE

A baby needs 52.3 calories for every pound per day. For example, a 7 lb. baby is being fed a brand of formula in which one spoonful = 40 calories.

7 lb. × 52.3 = 366 (calories needed per day)

366 ÷ 40 = 9 (spoonfuls of formula)

This baby needs 9 spoonfuls of formula per day. Each spoonful is diluted with 2 oz. of boiled water.

9 × 2 = 18 oz. per 24 hours.

If you feed the baby six meals per day (18 ÷ 6), each feeding should consist of 3 oz.

METRIC SYSTEM

A baby needs 115 calories for every kilogram per day. For example, a 3 kg. baby is being fed a brand of formula in which one spoonful = 40 calories.

3 kg. × 115 = 345 (calories needed per day)

345 ÷ 40 = 8.5 (spoonfuls of formula)

This baby needs 8.5 spoonfuls of formula per day. Each spoonful is diluted with 60 cc. of boiled water.

8.5 × 60 = 510 cc. per 24 hours

If you feed the baby six meals per day (510 ÷ 6), each feeding should consist of 85 cc.

The bottle must be heated up until it is lukewarm. You can test this by shaking a few drops on your wrist. It is permissible to do this on Shabbos as well. You can immerse the bottle in hot water that is in a "*keli sheni*" (a utensil that boiled water was poured into). However, the hot water should not cover the bottle completely. You may even put the baby's bottle into an empty utensil and pour hot water from a "*keli rishon*" (a utensil that the water was cooked in) directly on it, or you may put the bottle into a *keli rishon* that is no longer on the fire, if you are absolutely positive that the milk in the bottle will not reach the temperature of "*yad soledes bo*" (too hot to touch) — 45°C.[26]

Lactation Suppression

If you have chosen not to breast feed, then you will need to interrupt the natural process by which milk will be produced by the breasts. You need to notify your doctor and appropriate hospital staff members of your decision not to nurse in order to receive lactation suppression right after delivery.

Synthetic hormones are usually not recommended as they can cause thrombo-embolism (blood clots). However, another drug, Bromocriptine (Parlodel), causes the prolactin level to fall, thus inhibiting lactation. This drug can be administered hours after delivery and takes effect within 48 hours.

The breasts need to be bound by a tight-fitting bra or other binder. There should be absolutely no nursing or manual expression, as this would only stimulate the continued production of milk. Ice packs can be applied to sore breasts and an analgesic can be given to relieve discomfort.

If you do not breast feed, you can expect to begin to menstruate within six to eight weeks after delivery.

Nursing while Pregnant A woman who nurses while she is pregnant creates a situation in which nobody benefits. An opinion in the Gemara even allows a nursing mother to practice birth control in order to continue nursing. Rashi elaborates on this point, saying that the milk of a pregnant mother "dries up" and adversely affects the nursing baby.[27] (Consult your Rav for practical halachah.)

According to Dr. Chaim Yaffe, in addition to being an added drain on the resources of a pregnant woman, nursing during pregnancy increases the risk of miscarriage and may even diminish the nutritional potential available to the fetus.

If you become pregnant while nursing, you do not have to stop abruptly, but it is advisable to gradually wean your baby.

Nursing on Shabbos It is forbidden to express milk into a container on Shabbos.[28] In case of discomfort, however, it is permissible to express milk into anything that will not preserve the milk, such as the sink or a cloth (being careful not to squeeze the cloth). One may also express the milk into a container which contains a solvent that will render the milk unusable.[29]

It is preferable to express milk manually, but if this is too difficult one may use a hand pump. If a pump is used, one must either add an inedible solvent or empty the pump periodically so that the milk will not collect.[30]

It is permissible to express milk into the baby's mouth in order to encourage the baby to nurse.[31]

249 FEEDING YOUR
BABY

If for some reason the baby will not nurse or is separated from its mother whose milk is the baby's primary source of nourishment, it is permissible to express milk into a container in order to feed the baby. This applies even in cases where the baby has not yet become accustomed to mother's milk.[32]

Breast Care on Shabbos

If you need to use an ointment, you should smear the ointment on gauze pads (or nursing pads) before Shabbos. Then you may apply the prepared pads directly to the nipples on Shabbos, taking care not to rub in the ointment. Vitamin E oil can be allowed to drip onto the nipples without rubbing it in.[33]

Nursing on Yom Kippur

A nursing mother should make every effort to fast on Yom Kippur. However, if she needs to drink in order to maintain her milk supply (and fasting may cause her to temporarily lose her milk), she may drink less than a *shiur* on Yom Kippur.[34] If she started to fast and felt her milk supply dwindle during the fast, she should drink as much liquid as is required to restore the milk supply. This applies in the case of a very young infant, whose sole source of nourishment is nursing.

It is advisable for anyone to drink an extra amount of fluids the day before the fast, but this is especially true for the nursing mother. If the infant takes solids and fluids from another source, it is preferable to nurse as little as possible on Yom Kippur, substituting food and drink from other sources.

(For Tisha B'Av, see Chapter 7 on Fasting During Pregnancy. The same rules apply to the nursing mother.)

Milk and Honey

One of the blessings recited after the *haftarah* reading on Shabbos is also said at every Jewish wedding during the *sheva berachos* (the seven nuptial blessings). It is *"Mesame'ach Tzion b'vaneha* — Who makes Zion happy with her children." Eretz Yisrael has been called the "Mother of all of the People of Israel," for just as a child receives proper nutrition and care from his mother, so, too, the Jewish People receive the appropriate "spiritual nutrition" only in Eretz Yisrael.

The "Mother of all of the People of Israel" teaches us a very important lesson in childrearing. Most mothers attempt to fulfill their children's needs by nourishing them and providing them with "milk." Mothers gladly offer adequate educational opportunities and buy their children everything from baby shoes to wedding gowns, providing for their needs at every stage of life.

Eretz Yisrael adds another dimension to motherhood in regard to the care of the Jewish People. It is the land flowing with "milk and honey." Not only does it provide the nourishment of "milk," enabling each Jew to reach his full spiritual potential; it is also a land of "honey," which makes Torah life sweet as well as satisfying.

True "nursing" goes beyond the mechanical aspects of producing milk; true parenting goes beyond the fulfillment of basic needs. The "honey" component of mothering is essential as well. Throughout this book the notion that a mother is the guiding force in the spiritual growth of her entire household has been stressed. However, that's not all there is to it. A mother's mood and attitude can set the tone for the whole family. Torah without *simchah* — happiness — is not complete. To put it as simply as possible, a mother must make life sweet, enjoyable, and *fun.* For just as the Land of Israel makes life conducive to the spiritual development of her children while creating an atmosphere which is sweet and enjoyable, so, too, every Jewish mother, who provides the necessities of life in the form of milk to her children, should add honey and enhance the life of her children with "*simchas chayim* — the joy of life."

May every Jewish home be a Land of Milk and Honey.

NOTES

1. M. Eiger, S. Olds, *The Complete Book of Breastfeeding*, (Toronto: Bantam Books, 1972), p. 3.
2. N. Hacker, J. Moore, *Essentials of Obstetrics and Gynecology* (Philadelphia: W.B. Saunders, 1986).
3. J. Newman, M.D., *Infectious Disease Journal* (June 1987).
4. A. Cunningham, D. Jelliffe, and E. Jelliffe, "Breast-Feeding and Health in the 1980s: A Global Epidemiologic Review," *Journal of Pediatrics* 118:5 (May 1991), p. 664.
5. T. Abramov, *Straight from the Heart* (Jerusalem: Targum/Feldheim, 1990), p. 60.
6. M. Eiger, S. Olds, *The Complete Book of Breastfeeding*, p. 5.
7. *Sifri, Beha'alos'cha* 11:8.
8. *Kesubbos* 60a.
9. McCarthy, Van den Meer, *Midwife's Pregnancy and Childbirth Book* (Henry HOH & Co.)
10. *Ta'anis* 27b.
11. K. Niswander, A. Evans, eds., *Manual of Obstetrics* (Boston: Little, Brown & Co. 1991), p. 482.
12. N. Hacker, J. Moore, *Essentials of Obstetrics and Gynecology*, p. 100.
13. *Health Almanac, U.S. News and World Report*, June 1990.
14. *Bechoros* 7b.
15. Grossman, "The Effect of Post Partum Lactation Counseling on the Duration of Breast Feeding in Low Income Women," *American Journal of Disease in Children* 144, April 1990.
16. N. Hacker, J. Moore, *Essentials of Obstetrics and Gynecology*; Kamen and Kamen, *Total Nutrition for Breastfeeding Mothers* (Boston: Little, Brown & Co., 1986).
17. Kamen and Kamen, *Total Nutrition for Breastfeeding Mothers*.
18. *Yoma* 75a; *see* Rashi, *"Hallalu lo ta'amu"*; *see also* Sifri, *Beha'alos'cha* 11:8.
19. *Shulchan Aruch, Yoreh De'ah* 81:7; *see* Hebrew appendix.
20. *Berachos* 10.
21. *Vayikra Rabbah* 14.
22. *Gittin* 89a.
23. *Shulchan Aruch, Orach Chayim* 75:1; *Mishnah Berurah* 75:3.
24. *Shulchan Aruch* 75; *Mishnah Berurah* 75:5.
25. *Shulchan Aruch* 74:4, 75:1.
26. *Shemiras Shabbos K'hilchasah* 1:50.
27. *Kesubbos* 39.
28. *Shulchan Aruch, Orach Chayim* 328:34.

29. *Shulchan Aruch* 330:8; *Mishnah Berurah* 330:32; *see also* *Shemiras Shabbos K'hilchasah* 36:20.
30. *Shemiras Shabbos K'hilchasah* 36:20; *see* Hebrew appendix.
31. *Shulchan Aruch* 328:35; *Mishnah Berurah, Sha'ar Ha-Tziyun* 81.
32. *Shemiras Shabbos K'hilchasah* 36:21; *see* Hebrew appendix.
33. *Shulchan Aruch* 328:22.
34. *Shemiras Shabbos K'hilchasah* 39:17.

24 | Blessing Your Children

*'May Hashem turn His countenance upon
you' — at the time of prayer; 'and give
you peace' — peace is Torah.*

SIFRI ON BEMIDBAR 6:26

One of the most moving moments in parenthood is the
first time the parent blesses his newborn son or daughter on Shabbos eve. In some homes the father blesses
the children, and in some families the children receive
blessings from both the mother and the father.[1] We bless
both our young and grown children.[2]

Many people ask, "Who am I to bless my children? I
am not a great *tzaddik* or *talmid chacham*. Of what benefit could my blessing possibly be?"

The parent possesses an enormous power to confer
blessing upon his children. The Talmud says, "There are
three partners in man: the Holy One, Blessed Be He, his
father, and his mother."[3] Because the parent is considered *Hakadosh Baruch Hu*'s partner, when the father or
mother blesses the child, the blessing carries the force of
that of the third partner in the relationship — Hashem.

Some observe the custom of placing both hands on **Understanding**
the head of the child as they recite the *berachah*.[4] **the Blessing**
Others observe the custom of placing only the right
hand on the child's head; however, once the child is

married, the parent places both hands on the child's head so as to include a blessing for the child's spouse as well.[5]

The blessing is composed of two parts. The first part has two forms, feminine and masculine. For a girl we say,

יְשִׂמֵךְ אֱלֹקִים כְּשָׂרָה רִבְקָה רָחֵל וְלֵאָה.

"May Hashem establish you like Sarah, Rivkah, Rachel and Leah."

For a boy, we say,

יְשִׂמְךָ אֱלֹקִים כְּאֶפְרַיִם וְכִמְנַשֶּׁה.

"May Hashem establish you like Efrayim and Menashe."

The second part is the same for both genders:

יְבָרֶכְךָ ה' וְיִשְׁמְרֶךָ.

יָאֵר ה' פָּנָיו אֵלֶיךָ, וִיחֻנֶּךָּ.

יִשָּׂא ה' פָּנָיו אֵלֶיךָ, וְיָשֵׂם לְךָ שָׁלוֹם.

"May Hashem bless you and protect you. May His countenance shine upon you and be gracious to you. May Hashem turn His countenance upon you and give you peace" (Bemidbar 6:24-26).

Invoking the example of the Matriarchs seems natural for our daughters. But why is it that we do not use the same formula for our sons, exhorting them to be like our Patriarchs, Avraham, Yitzchak and Ya'akov? Why do we instead confer the blessing that they should be like Efrayim and Menashe, the sons of Yosef?

The simple answer can be found in Ya'akov Avinu's introduction to this blessing. He addressed Efrayim and Menashe, saying that "Israel will use you as a blessing."[6]

To understand why Ya'akov exchanged the Patriarchs with Efrayim and Menashe, we must look into the backgrounds of the people involved. Efrayim and Menashe, it seems, had one thing in common with the Matriarchs that the Patriarchs did not. All of the Matriarchs were

great, righteous women, but they hailed from the homes
of wicked people — what we call today "a bad environment." Of our forefathers, only Avraham came from a
house of idol worship. Yitzchak and Ya'akov were raised
in the homes of great *tzaddikim*. Efrayim and Menashe
were similar to the Matriarchs in that they were raised in
the immoral environment of Egypt. Even though their father was Yosef the Righteous, he was also the viceroy of
Egypt. Could he really give them enough to compensate
for friendships and a culture steeped in immorality?

Efrayim and Menashe reached a high level of piety,
and, like the Matriarchs, achieved this against all odds.
They were *tzaddikim* despite their environment.

There is a well-known Yiddish expression: "*Kleine
kinder, kleine tzores; grosse kinder, grosse tzores* —
Small children, small problems; big children, big problems." Small children make tremendous demands on a
parent's time and energy. Often we feel overwhelmed by
the physical demands of constant giving, especially
when our sleep is disturbed. But ask any parent of teen-
age children, and they will confirm that the problems involved in raising small children seem insignificant in comparison to the anguish of seeing one's child grow rebellious. Having a child who abandons the Torah is the
greatest fear of a Jewish parent.

Our efforts as educators are limited in their ability to
have a long-term effect. Although we must toil to educate our children, there are no assurances. As our children mature, we begin to lose the complete control we
previously had over their behavior. A certain amount of
mazal is needed to make our educational efforts succeed.[7]

External influences can have a strong impact upon
our children. We cannot always guarantee that our children will not be exposed to a negative environment. We
therefore give both our sons and daughters the blessing
that they should be like those *tzaddikim* who were not
tempted by their immoral surroundings and maintained

their ethical and righteous behavior. We pray that they will be proud of the Torah way of life and observe the mitzvos. No matter what environment they are exposed to, we bless them that they should be like Sarah, Rivkah, Rachel, Leah, Efrayim and Menashe. And Hashem should protect them and give them peace.

NOTES

1. *Be'er Heitev* 262:2; and it is written there that the reason can be found in the writings of the Ari z"l.
2. *Siddur Beis Ya'akov*, customs of Friday night.
3. *Niddah* 31a.
4. *Siddur Beis Ya'akov*, customs of Friday night.
5. *Otzar Dinim u'Minhagim, Birkas Ha-Banim*, p. 56, in the name of *Pachad Yitzchak*; see also *Kaf Ha-Chayim* 262:16, for more customs during the blessings.
6. *Bereshis* 48:20.
7. *Mo'ed Katan* 28a.

25 | A Look Ahead

*As soon as a baby begins to talk, his
father speaks to him in Hebrew and
teaches him Torah.*
SIFRI, PARASHAS EKEV

The first year of life is one of spectacular growth, development and change. Though every baby is unique, there are specific developmental tasks which are accomplished within a set period of time. Parents can certainly contribute to the optimal advancement of their baby's potential, but they must accept the pace that their baby establishes for himself.

Other than for a few colds, your baby, God willing, should see the doctor only for well-baby checkups. These are usually scheduled at age 2-6 weeks, 6 months, and one year. It is a good idea to write down any questions you have before you see the doctor, so you do not forget what you wanted to ask.

During the first 15-18 months of life, your baby will **Immunizations** receive his immunizations. These immunizations are actually a series of inoculations given at different monthly intervals (see schedule below). Vaccinating your child is an important, responsible way to prevent many life-threatening diseases. Although reactions to inoculations can occur, the immunological benefits of vaccinating your children far outweigh any possible reaction.

DTP

The diphtheria-tetanus-pertussis vaccine is a three-in-one immunization, which is administered intramuscularly in the thigh area.

Though one rarely hears of people contracting diphtheria, cases still are reported each year. Due to widespread immigration throughout the world, a child must be vaccinated against this deadly disease.

The tetanus toxoid immunizes a child against tetanus, which is a potentially fatal infection caused by an aerobic bacteria, clostridium tetani. Transmission occurs by means of puncture wounds and burns.

The pertussis component of DTP is a vaccination against whooping cough. Children under the age of two who have not been immunized are especially vulnerable to this highly contagious disease, which continues to take young lives even in modern times. There can be slight fever and irritability after vaccination. However, investigators in a British National Childhood Encephalopathy Study (NCES) found that it is very rare for the pertussis vaccine to result in acute neurological illness (1:140,000), and most reactions are temporary.[1]

Not all children have a reaction. For those who do, Dr. Erlichman recommends: Within half an hour of a DTP injection, give one acetaminophen (Tylenol/Acamol) suppository, and another later in the evening. Tepid baths will relieve fever and raise spirits. An alcohol compress will relieve swelling at the injection site. If your child's temperature rises above 102.2°F (39°C), or if he continues to cry hysterically or exhibit extreme sleepiness, seek medical attention at once.

Acetaminophen (Tylenol/Acamol) should be administered according to the weight of your child as per the following specifications:

For Suppository: 20 mg./2.2 lb. (1 kg.)
For Syrup: 1 cc./2.2 lb. (1 kg.) (125 mg. = 5 cc./1 tsp.)

POLIO

Two types of polio vaccines are used. Sabin, or oral TOPV, is administered either by drops applied directly on the tongue or on a sugar cube. Since it contains attenuated living organisms which stimulate the formation of antibodies, for a few days after the vaccination the baby's soiled (bowel movement) diapers must be carefully wrapped in a bag before disposal. This should be followed by scrupulous handwashing. The Salk vaccine is administered by subcutaneous injection in the arm. There are no reactions to either polio vaccine.

MENINGITIS

The meningitis vaccine is an important addition to the immunization schedule. Referred to as HIB or HbCV, it protects against the most common form of meningitis, haemophilus influenzae. The reaction to this vaccine is usually in the form of localized swelling at the injection site.

VIRAL HEPATITIS

As of January 1, 1992, all children born in Israel are vaccinated against Hepatitis B, which is considered more serious than Hepatitis A, because it can result in life-threatening, irreversible damage to the liver. The Ministry of Health decided to implement this vaccine in the immunization schedule to prevent the need for liver transplants, which are often required after severe liver damage. This vaccine is administered by subcutaneous injection in the arm. There is no reaction, other than slight swelling at the injection site.

MMR

The measles-mumps-rubella (German measles) vaccine is a three-in-one immunization against these three diseases. It is injected subcutaneously in the arm. Reaction to the MMR is usually delayed until 5-12 days after the vaccination. The baby might get a rash and slightly elevated temperature for no more than 24 hours. In the event of a measles epidemic, the age of innoculation may be lowered from 15 months to 12 months.

Schedule of Immunizations

U.S.A.*	ISRAEL
2 months DTP TOPV (Sabin) HbCV	**at birth** viral hepatitis B vaccine (HBV) **1 month** viral hepatitis B vaccine
4 months DTP TOPV HbCV	**2 months** DTP polio vaccine (Salk) HbCV
6 months DTP HbCV	**4 months** DTP polio vaccine (Salk) TOPV (Sabin) HbCV
15 months MMR HbCV	**6 months** DTP TOPV (Sabin) viral hepatitis B vaccine HIB
18 months DTP booster TOPV booster	**12 months** DTP booster polio vaccine (Salk) TOPV (Sabin) HbCV
* Recommended by the American Academy of Pediatrics	**15 months** MMR

DTP: diphtheria-tetanus-pertussis
HbCV/HIB: haemophilus influenzae B (meningitis vaccine)
MMR: measles-mumps-rubella
TOPV: trivalent oral polio vaccine

Parenthood is not just a one-way giving/teaching **Learn from** relationship. We can also learn from our children, **Your Baby** even while they are very young.

The story is told of Reb Zusha from Avipoli, who was one of the disciples of the Maggid of Mezritch. Twice a year, winter and summer, he would go to his Rebbe and stay for two or three months. He felt that he needed to absorb as much wisdom as possible to sustain him during the long periods he would be away from his Rebbe.

Once when Reb Zusha came to his Rebbe, he was immediately told to return home that same day. Although he did not understand, Reb Zusha was willing to follow his Rebbe's command. However, he requested that his Rebbe give him some *tzeidah la-derech* — some spiritual nourishment to sustain him along the way.

"I will teach you something that will give you a great deal of insight," said the Maggid. "Observe a baby and learn from him three basic attributes:

1. a baby is never idle;

2. when a baby wants something, he cries to his parent; and

3. a baby is always happy."

NOTE

1. K.R. Wentz, E.K. Marcuse, "Diphtheria-Tetanus-Pertussis Vaccine and Serious Neurological Illness: An Updated Review," *Pediatrics* 87:3 (March 1991), p. 287.

26 | Giving Gold

Why did Hashem command Moshe to teach the women first? In order that they should guide their children to Torah.

SHEMOS RABBAH 28

A young couple who had just been blessed with a baby approached the Chafetz Chayim to ask when they should begin the education process of their child. The Chafetz Chayim surprised them with his answer: "You should have begun nine months ago!"

Although the mitzvah of educating children is actually fulfilled years after their birth, it is important to prepare oneself emotionally and spiritually for this lofty, difficult and time-consuming task. The primary goal of a parent is to raise children to become God-fearing Jews. For this reason, as soon as the birth of your baby is announced, you will receive the following blessing from friends and family: "May you merit raising your son/ daughter to Torah, *chuppah* (the marriage canopy) and *ma'asim tovim* (good deeds)."

On One Foot A potential convert once came to Shammai and asked to be taught all of the Torah while standing on one foot, in other words in capsulized form. As Shammai truly understood the great depth and breadth of Torah thought, he knew this was an impossible task, and so he threw the potential convert out of his home. The man then approached Hillel with the same request. Hillel answered, "Whatever you find distasteful, do not do to others." In that short sentence, Hillel summarized the Commandments that apply in matters between man and his fellow man. He then instructed the man as follows: "This is the essence of Torah — the rest is commentary. Now, go study the commentary," and educate yourself in the practical implementation of this great principle.[1]

Although this book deals mainly with pregnancy and childbirth, we should also like to convey — "on one foot," so to speak — a few brief, basic principles of educating children. For as the Chafetz Chayim suggested, even at this early stage one should be concerned with this mitzvah.

Investment is the most appropriate description of a parent's obligation in educating his child. Education does not require sacrifice, which implies giving up one thing in order to attain something else. Rather, it demands investment — depositing one's efforts in order to reap benefit. One must invest both money and time in one's children.

Investing Money

A parent must pay for schools, teachers and books, but we are assured that we will be reimbursed for all these expenses. Each year a family is allotted a certain amount of money by Hashem, but this does not include the expenses of teaching children Torah. For this expense, the more you spend, the more Hashem will give you.[2] You will not incur a loss, no matter how much you spend. Instead, you will rear and be blessed with a child who will sanctify God's Name.

Investing Time

Fathers are commanded to spend time learning with their children, as it is written, "V'limadetem osam es beneichem — You should teach [words of Torah] to your children."[3] This commandment applies first and foremost to your own child.[4]

Just as important as actively teaching your children

Torah is the passive instruction given by your example. Children are greatly influenced by what they see in the home. The home environment can have a more enduring effect on their commitment to Divine service than can their peer groups, schools and books. When a child observes his mother dressed modestly, his father going to shul, charity being given, and family members refraining from speaking *lashon ha-ra*, it makes a deep impression on his heart and in his soul. Lighting Chanukah candles, sitting together at the *Seder*, hearing *berachos* recited, and singing at the Shabbos table are all links in a chain connecting the parents and the child with the Almighty.

The power of example certainly applies to learning Torah. If a son sees his father waste time, one should not be surprised when the son seeks other diversions instead of learning. It is not likely that this child, who is merely following his father's example, will ever succeed as a Torah scholar. On the other hand, if a son sees that his father regularly schedules time for learning Torah, he will want to emulate his father and spend his time learning Torah as well. He will readily accept the fact that learning Torah is the natural thing to do with one's time.

Immediately following the command to learn and teach — "*V'shinnantam l'vanecha* — And you should diligently teach your children," the Torah says, "*V'dibarta bam* — And you should speak in them [words of Torah]."[5] The following may be learned from the juxtaposition of these two commands: "Teach your children" — how? "Speak in them" — in words of Torah. When your child sees you "speaking in them," i.e., being involved in Torah, he will learn to love Torah as you do. In this way one diligently teaches his children.

The mother plays a great role in her children's education. For although she is not commanded to actively teach her children Torah, she certainly has the obligation to imbue her home with an atmosphere that is conducive to spiritual growth. Her specific responsibility is to prepare her children to learn, and to take them to school. For this, the Sages tell us, she earns an even greater reward than the father.[6]

Of course, the mother and father should work together in order to establish their home as a microcosmic Sanctuary.

The Holy Ark, the *Aron Ha-Kodesh*, was one of the primary vessels in the *Beis Hamikdash.* On the Ark were the *keruvim* — two angelic, child-like figures **The Golden Keruvim** which faced one another. Their wings were spread over the Ark, and Hashem spoke through them, teaching words of Torah to Moshe.

According to *halachah*, the vessels of the *Beis Hamikdash* were to be made of gold. However, if they could not be made of gold, they could also be made of a less precious metal. The exception to this rule was the *keruvim*, for they could be fashioned only from gold. No other metal was acceptable. The reason given for this is the human appearance of the *keruvim* and their location in the Holy of Holies — gentiles and heretics could claim that the *keruvim* were a form of idol worship. Thus the specific stipulation that the *keruvim* had to be made exactly as commanded in the Torah, "And you should make two golden *keruvim.*"[7]

Another interpretation may be applied on the level of *derash.* Our Sages tell us that the Ark represents the Torah. Thus the two child-like faces represent *tinokos shel beis rabban* — young children learning Torah with their teachers. The lesson learned from the two *keruvim* that face each other is that we should teach the Torah in a way that the children will be figuratively facing one another, caring for one another: "*U'feneihem ish el achiv.*"[8] This is a teaching of loving-kindness, altruistic rather than egoistic. Its ultimate goal is to help others, build friendships and strengthen society through Torah that is *Toras Chesed.*

The halachic stipulation that the *keruvim* had to be made from gold is a lesson to us that when it comes to educating our children there can be no "second best," no compromises. We can fulfill other mitzvos by using less than the best material, but not the mitzvah of educating our children. For that we are obligated to provide only the best, only gold.

Investing gold in our children will produce golden children. Just as gold will always come out of the fire unscathed and unchanged,[9] so too will our golden children have the strength and spirit to confront the fires of physical and spiritual peril and emerge pure. They will shine like gold and spread their wings like the *keruvim* to protect the Ark of the Torah.[10]

May we merit that Hashem will speak through our children, as they grow to become the future teachers of Torah. And may it be in Eretz Yisrael. For on the verse describing the rivers that went out from Eden, "the first...encompasses the whole land...where there is gold; and the gold of that land is good,"[11] *Chazal* say, "*Where there is gold* — 'gold' means words of Torah. *And the gold of that land is good* — this teaches that there is no Torah like the Torah of Eretz Yisrael, and no wisdom like the wisdom of Eretz Yisrael."[12] And may it be in Yerushalayim, "For from *Tzion* will go forth Torah and the word of Hashem from Yerushalayim."[13]

כִּי מִצִּיּוֹן תֵּצֵא תוֹרָה וּדְבַר ה' מִירוּשָׁלָיִם.

NOTES

1. *Shabbos* 31a.
2. *Beitzah* 16a.
3. *Devarim* 11:19.
4. *Kiddushin* 30a; Rambam on *Talmud Torah*, ch. 1, halachos 2-3; *Shulchan Aruch, Yoreh De'ah* 245:1.
5. *Devarim* 6:7.
6. *Berachos* 17a.
7. *Mechilta, Parashas Yisro* 20:20, Os 3.

8. *Shemos* 25:20.
9. *Bemidbar Rabbah* 12.
10. And so it is written in *Bereshis* 3:24: "He placed at the east of the Garden of Eden the *keruvim* and their flaming sword...to guard the tree of life." And *Chazal* say that the tree of life is Torah (*Berachos* 32b).
11. *Bereshis* 2:11,12.
12. *Bereshis Rabbah* 16:4.
13. *Yeshayahu* 2:3.

Appendices

WARNING SIGNS DURING PREGNANCY

Though every woman should expect her pregnancy to proceed normally, God willing, occasionally a pregnant woman might experience symptoms which require an immediate consultation with a doctor.

Bleeding: any bleeding, no matter how slight.

Abdominal Pain: persistent cramping, stabbing pains, or a dull ache.

Vomiting: persistent or forceful vomiting accompanied by weakness or fever.

Illness: fever or frequent diarrhea.

Urinary Disturbances: a burning sensation or pain during urination, sometimes accompanied by pain in the side or lower back.

Leg Pains: pain, redness, swelling, and/or sensation of heat in the calf area of the leg.

Reduction of Fetal Movements: from week 28 any reduction or change (lessening) in the charateristics or frequency of fetal movements.

Edema; Visual Disturbances: swelling of the hands or face, severe headache, blurred vision or other visual problems.

Watery Discharge: any sudden flow of fluid from the vagina.

APPENDIX B:

BREAST SELF-EXAMINATION

The responsibility to care for our bodies extends beyond health maintenance to disease prevention. The average woman has one chance in ten of developing breast cancer during her lifetime, and it is the leading cause of death in women aged 39-44.[1] Most lumps have been found by women themselves while examining their bodies, and eight out of ten lumps are benign (non-cancerous). Early detection and treatment offer the best chances for a healthy outcome.[2] In fact, most women treated for early breast cancer will be free from breast cancer for the rest of their lives.

All women, therefore, should learn the simple procedures of breast care: monthly breast self-examination, routine examination by a health professional, and regular mammograms after the age of 40.

Breast self-examination is most effectively done 2-3 days after the end of your period. A woman who has stopped menstruating should choose the same day each month to examine herself. The idea behind self-examination is to get a feeling for what is "normal" for you, so that you will be able to distinguish any suspicious changes.

The National Cancer Institute suggests these 6 steps in performing a breast self-examination:

1. Stand before a mirror. Inspect both breasts for anything unusual, such as any discharge from the nipples or puckering, dimpling, or scaling of the skin.

2. Watching closely in the mirror, clasp your hands behind your head and press your hands forward.

3. Next, press your hands firmly on your hips and bow slightly towards your mirror as you pull your shoulders and elbows forward.

4. Raise your left arm. Use three or four fingers of your right hand to explore your left breast firmly, care-

fully and thoroughly. Beginning at the outer edge, press the flat part of your fingers in small circles, moving the circles slowly around the breast. Gradually work toward the nipple. Be sure to cover the entire breast. Pay special attention to the area between the breast and the underarm, including the underarm itself. Feel for any unusual lump or mass under the skin.

5. Gently squeeze the nipple and look for a discharge. (If you have any discharge during the month — whether or not it is during breast self-examination — see your doctor.) Repeat steps 4 and 5 on your right breast.

6. Steps 4 and 5 should be repeated lying down. Lie flat on your back with your left arm over your head and a pillow or folded towel under your left shoulder. This position flattens the breast and makes it easier to examine. Use the same circular motion described earlier. Repeat the exam on your right breast.[3]

Ask a doctor or other health professional to review with you the steps of breast self-examination to assure that you have learned the proper procedure. Be alert to any changes in your breast, and be prepared to discuss those changes promptly with your doctor.

Establish a relationship with an appropriate health care professional, and have your breasts examined annually. By age 40, all women should have had a baseline mammogram (breast x-ray), with follow-up mammograms every 1-2 years.

Remember, only through our awareness and diligence can this disease be promptly detected and treated.

BREAST SELF-EXAM DURING PREGNANCY

Before pregnancy and after the cessation of nursing you can routinely examine your breasts. During pregnancy and lactation, the breasts undergo many structural changes. Performing the breast self-examination during these times, therefore, is not effective. Your obstetrician can best differentiate between enlarged milk ducts and possible growths.

NOTES

1. H. Barber, D. Fields, S. Kaufman, *OB/GYN Procedures* (Philadelphia: Lippincott, 1990), p. 419.
2. National Cancer Institute, National Institute of Health Publication No. 90-2000, June 1988.
3. Reprinted with permission from the National Cancer Institute.

RDA NUTRITION CHART

The U.S. Federal Food and Drug Administration suggests the amount of nutrients needed on a daily basis to keep people healthy. This unit of measurement is called Recommended Daily Allowance (RDA).

U.S. RDAs for Adults and Children over Age Four

gr.= grams; IU= international units; mg.= milligrams; mcg.= micrograms

Nutrient	U.S. RDA	In Pregnancy
Protein	44 gr.	+ 30 gr.
Vitamin A	5000 IU	+ 1250 IU
Vitamin D	400 IU	+ 400 IU
Vitamin E	8 mg.	+ 2 mg.
Vitamin C	60 mg.	+ 20 mg.
Thiamine (B_1)	1 mg.	+ 0.4 mg.
Riboflavin (B_2)	1.2 mg.	+ 0.3 mg.
Niacin	15 mg.	+ 2 mg.
Calcium	1200 mg.	+ 400 mg.
Iron	18 mg.	+ 30-60 mg.
Vitamin B_6 (pyridoxine)	2 mg.	+ 0.6 mg.
Folic Acid	0.4 mg.	+ 0.4 mg.
Vitamin B_{12}	3 mcg.	+ 1 mcg.
Phosphorus	1 gr.	+ 400 mg.
Iodine	150 mcg.	+ 25 mcg.
Magnesium	300 mg.	+ 150 mg.
Zinc	15 mg.	+ 5 mg.

APPENDIX D:

A NOTE ABOUT TAY-SACHS DISEASE

Tay-Sachs is an autosomal recessive inherited disease in which an infant lacks the enzyme hexosaminidase A. This enzyme is necessary for lipid (fat) metabolism. Without hexosaminidase A, fat deposits accumulate on nerve cells, gradually destroying them. The newborn appears normal at birth but his condition progressively deteriorates, resulting in blindness, paralysis and death by 3-5 years of age.

In an autosomal recessive inherited disease, when one parent is a carrier of the defective gene, 50% of the children can inherit the carrier status, but none will be affected by the disease. However, if *both* parents are carriers, then 25% of the offspring are likely to have the disease, 50% will be carriers, and 25% will be unaffected.

Tay-Sachs disease is a tragedy that in many cases can be avoided. It is often recommended that young people in their late teens or early adulthood before marriage undergo a simple blood test to screen for Tay-Sachs. Since the disease only occurs in the offspring of *two* carrier parents, those who know they carry the defective gene should not marry other carriers.

Today, many Rabbinic authorities advocate Tay-Sachs screening before marriage. In the United States, you can contact your local County Health Service for information about where one can be tested. In Israel, screening is done through the Ministry of Health and through the various health fund clinics.

מקורות והערות

פרק 1

1. מתוך הספר אני מאמין (עמ' 93, הוצאת מוסד הרב קוק).
2. שמות א', ט"ז, ועיין בפירושו של התורה תמימה.
3. רש"י שם י"ז.
4. שם י"ט, ופירש האבן עזרא: "כי חיות הנה'": - כח חיים הרבה יש להם".
5. סוטה י"ב, א'.
6. ראה רש"י, שמות ל"ח, ח' ד"ה "במראת הצבאת".
7. ראה רש"ן ורמב"ן בראשית ט', ז'.
8. בראשית רבה ט', ז': "רבי נחמן בר שמואל בשם רב שמואל בר נחמן אמר 'הנה טוב מאוד' זה יצר טוב, 'והנה טוב מאוד' זה יצר רע, וכי יצר הרע טוב מאוד, אתמהא, אלא שאלולי יצר הרע לא בנה אדם בית ולא נשא אשה ולא הוליד ולא נשא ונתן, וכן שלמה אומר (קהלת ד') "כי היא קנאת איש מרעהו".
9. בכורות מ"ה, א'.

פרק 2

3. רש"י במסכת יומא מ"ז, א', ד"ה "איכא דאמרי בשכבת זרע" וז"ל "קאמר שאין יצירת הוולד מכל הטיפה אלא מן הבירור שבה. זרד לשון חבילי זרדים טודי"ל כלומר בירור טיפה שקלטה אמי הזרד גבר ועלה לגג." והמקור לדברי רש"י הוא הגמ' במסכת נדה ל"א, א'.
6. נדה ל"ח, א'. 271 ימים לאחר שהזרע נקלט, אבל לפעמים לא נקלט ביום הראשון ונקלט רק ביום השני או השלישי.
8. סוטה ב', א'.
9. רמ"א שו"ע יורה דעה סי' רמ"ב סע' ל"א וראה ש"ד ס"ק מ"ט.

פרק 3

4. יומא פ"ה, א': "דתניא מהיכן הולד נוצר, מראשו שנאמר 'ממעי אמי אתה גוזי' (תהלים ע"א) ואומר 'גזי נזרך והשליכי' (ירמיה ז', כ"ט) ואבא שאול אומר מטיבורו ומשלח שרשיו אילך ואילך". וראה ירושלמי נדה פרק ג' הלכה ג'.
8. נדה ל', א' משנה שם: "רבי ישמעאל אומר יום מ"א תשב לזכר ולנדה יום פ"א תשב לזכר ולנקבה ולנדה, שהזכר נגמר למ"א והנקבה לפ"א, וחכ"א אחד בריית הזכר ואחד בריית הנקבה זה וזה מ"א."

פרק 4

1. ראה רמב"ם פירוש המשניות, פסחים פרק רביעי משנה י'.
2. רמב"ן ויקרא כ"ו, י"א.
3. ברכי יוסף יורה דעה סי' של"ו ס"ק ב' וז"ל "נראה דהאידנא אין לו לסמוך על הנס. וחייב החולה להתנהג בדרך העולם לקרוא לרופא שירפאנו ולא כל כמיניה לשנות סוגיין דעלמא ואין לו רשות לשנות דרך העולם ולומר כי הוא גדול מכמה חסידי הדורות שנתרפאו על ידי הרופאים. וכמעט איסור יש בדבר, אי משום יוהרא ואי משום לסמוך אניסא במקום סכנה ולהזכיר עוונותיו בשעת חוליו. אמנם ינהג כדרך של בני אדם וארחת כל ארעא להתרפאות על ידי רופא ולבו בל עמו רק ידבק בקונו למתקף ברחמי בכל לבו ובו יבטח דוקא."
4. שבט יהודה על השו"ע יו"ד ס' של"ו וז"ל "ענין בקשת הרופא הוא דבר מוכרח ויש לו עיקר מן התורה וכמעט שיש חיוב על החולה והקרובים לחזר על הרופא המובהק ולחזר אחר הסממנין המועילין לרפאות אותו חולי. וכל המתעצל ומתרשל בדבר זה ולא יחוש על הרפואה בדרך הטבע אלא יסמוך על דרך הנס לומר שהקב"ה ישלח דברו וירפאהו בחנם אין זה אלא מן המתמיהין ודעת שוטים היא זו וקרוב הוא להיות פושע בעצמו ועתיד ליתן את הדין...."
5. מדרש שמואל פרשה ד'.
6. חזון איש קובץ איגרות ח"א איגרת קל"ו.
7. סנהדרין י"ז, ב'.
8. ראש השנה כ"ט, א', ראה מאמרו של ד"ר אברהם שטיינברג "יחס ההלכה לרפואה" בספר אסיא ח"ו עמ' 9.
9. כתב הנודע ביהודה יו"ד סי' ק"כ "מה שאמרו אי אפשר לפתיחת הקבר בלא דם אין חילוק בין גרם הפתיחה הוא מבפנים ובין גרם הפתיחה הוא מבחוץ שהרופא הכניס אצבעו או איזה כלי ופתח פי המקור" עכ"ל, ופוסקים רבים דחו את דבריו וביניהם הרב ברוך פרנקל זצ"ל בהגהותיו על הנודע ביהודה וכן החכמת אדם בבינת אדם סי' כ"ג וחת"ס בסי' קע"ט והובאו בפתחי תשובה סי' קצ"ד ס"ק ד'. וכן החזו"א ביו"ד סי' פ"ג דחה את דבריו. ועיין בספר טהרת הבית ח"ב של הגר"ע יוסף במשמרת הטהרה עמ' דף נ"ה שהאריך מאד בנושא, ומסיק להלכה דיש להקל אפילו אם נפתח המקור ע"י הכלי. ואין צורך להאריך בנידון זה מכיון שהספקולים אינו פותח את המקור, לכן אין שום חשש שמא תראה דם, והיא טהורה אף ללא בדיקה.
10. כך הורה לי הגר"מ אליהו.
13. שו"ת אגרות משה חשן משפט ח"ב סי' ע"א.
14. שו"ת ציץ אליעזר חי"ד סי' ק"א.
18. כך הורה לי הגר"מ אליהו.

פרק 5

2. שו"ע יו"ד סי' קפ"ט סע' ל"ג, ובכל זאת ממשיכה לחשוש מאותו יום לעונה בינונית בלבד עוד פעמיים, דהיינו ביום השישים וביום התשעים (דרכי טהרה עמוד פ"ד).

3. שו"ת רעק"א סי' קכ"ח וכן פסק הרב משה פיינשטיין ז"ל בתשובות
המודפסות בסוף ספר "הלכות נדה" של הרב ש' איידר וכן נפסק להלכה
בספר טהרת הבית ח"א עמ' פ"א - פ"ד.

4. שו"ע שם.

5. בראשית כ"א, א'.

6. רש"י שם.

7. יבמות ס"ד, א'.

8. בראשית כ"ה, כ"ב.

9. ספר הזכרון על פירוש רש"י (לרבי אברהם בקראט. [ממגורשי ספרד]).

10. בראשית ל', ב'.

פרק 6

15. דברים כ', י"ט.

16. רמב"ם הל' אבל פ' י"ד הל' כ"ג וכ"ד.

17. שבת קכ"ט א': "בל תשחית דגופאי עדיף לי" והובא ברי"ף במקום.

18. שערי תשובה שער ג' פרק פ"ב.

19. הלכות דעות פרק ד' הל' א', ועיין עוד בקונטרס "העישון בהלכה" של הרב
מנחם סליי שדן באריכות בביאור השיטות השונות.

20. שו"ע חושן משפט סי' תכ"ז, שו"ת אג"מ חושן משפט ח"ב סי' ע"ו.

21. ערוך השולחן חושן משפט סי' תכ"ז סע"ח'.

22. באר הגולה חושן משפט סוף סי' תכ"ז.

23. "דעו כי שלמות הגוף קודמת לשלמות הנפש והיא כמפתח הפותח
טרקלין, ולכן עיקר כוונת מוסר על שלמות גופכם ותקון מדותיכם לפתוח
לפניכם דלתות שמיים" - - אגרת המוסר של הרמב"ם לבנו רבי אברהם
(מודפס בהקדמת הספר "איסור העישון בהלכה"). וראה גם מאמרו של הרב
אפרים וינברג, "שמירת החיים והבריאות בהלכה", בצומת התורה
והמדינה, חלק ג'. וראה אנציקלופדיה הלכתית רפואית חלק א', ד"ר אברהם
שטיינברג ערך "בריאות".

פרק 7

1. שו"ע או"ח סי' תרי"ז סע' א'.

2. עיין בשו"ת רדב"ז ח"ג (תמ"ד). ששם כתב בשם הר"ן דאדם שנצטוה
לאכל ביו"כ ואינו מציית לעצת הרופאים והוא צם אין זה מידת חסידות.
אדרבה הרי הוא שופך דמים. ואפילו לפי דעת האחרונים שאמרו דמי שהיה
דינו יעבור ואל יהרג ולא עבר הרי הוא במחיצות הצדיקים, ושלא כדעת
הרמב"ם ז"ל, מ"מ ה"ה במקום דאיכא קידוש השם שמסר עצמו על דתו
ית', אבל מי שהוא חולה שיש בו סכנה אמדוהו לאכול יש לו לאכול ואפילו
על הספק ע"כ. ועיין בשו"ת בציץ אליעזר ח"י סי' כ"ה פרק י"ד. ובשו"ת יחוה
דעת ח"א סי' ס"א.

3. תורת היולדת פרק נ' סי' ד', וכן שמעתי מהגרח"פ שיינברג.

4. ערוך השולחן סי' תרי"ח סע' א'. וכן שם סי' תקנ"ד סע' ז'.

5. שו"ת איגרות משה או"ח ח"ד סי' קכ"א.

6. לפי הוראות ד"ר חיים יפה, ראש מחלקת נשים, ביה"ח "בקור חולים", וכן
הורה לי הלכה למעשה הגרח"פ שיינברג.

7. שו"ת ארץ צבי לגאון הרב אריה צבי פראמער זצ"ל סימן פ"ח ושו"ת אג"מ
או"ח ח"ג סי' צ"א. ועיין עוד בשו"ת ציץ אליעזר ח"י סי' כ"ה פרק כ"ב.

8. שו"ע או"ח סי' תרי"ז סע' ב', ועיין במ"ב וכה"ח שם לפרטי הדינים.

9. כן שמעתי מהגרח"פ שיינברג.

10. שו"ע או"ח סי' תק"נ סע' א' ובמ"ב ס"ק ג', וסי' תקנ"ד סע' ה'. ועל אף
שהרמ"א בסי' תק"נ כתב שנהגו להחמיר פסק הערה"ש בסי' תקנ"ד סע' ז'
שלא יחמירו על עצמן. וכן כתב בשו"ת יחוה דעת ח"א סי' ל"ה שבזמן הזה
ירדה חולשה לעולם, גם לבנות אשכנז יש להקל.

11. ערוך השולחן סי' תק"נ סע' א'.

12. רמ"א סי' תק"נ סע' א', וכתב הדרכי משה בסי' תקנ"ד אות ג' שזה המנהג
ולא כמו שפסק רבינו ירוחם בנתיב כ"ז בשם הגאונים שמעוברת אסורה
להתענות אפילו אם אינה מצטערת זולתי בט"ב ויה"כ משום צער הולד.
וכתב הערוך השולחן בסי' תק"נ סי' א' שבג' צומות מעוברת רשאית
להתענות אם היא חזקה. וע"ע בשו"ת יחוה דעת ח"א סי' ל"ה שפסק שאסור
להן להחמיר על עצמן.

13. שו"ת יחוה דעת חלק א' סי' ל"ה.

14. שו"ת או"ח סי' תקנ"ד סע' ה'.

15. טור או"ח בשם הרמב"ן, סי' תקנ"ד. ערוך השולחן סי' תקנ"ד סע' ז'.

16. ספר תורת היולדת פרק מ"ח הע' ח' הביא בשם ספר אבילות החורבן
שנהגו להקל במקומות החמים משום שבאו לידי סכנה, כ"כ הג"ר צדקה
אב"ד בגדד. וכן הובאה דעתו בשו"ת יחוה דעת ח"א סי' מ"ב. ועיין בשו"ת
ציץ אליעזר חלק י"ז סי' כ' אות ד'.

17. מדובר באופן שיש לו סיבה טובה לחשוש, כגון שבעבר היו לה הפלות או
לידות מוקדמות מהצפוי, או שהיא חלשה ביותר, או שעליה להיות בשמירת
הריון וכדומה. ואם עליה לאכול פחות, פחות מכשיעור, עיין במה שכתבנו
בהערה 20, ותשאל שאלת חכם.

18. וכן כתב בספר מועדים וזמנים ח"ז סי' רנ"ב בשם הגאון מבריסק. ערוך
השולחן סי' תקנ"ד סע' ז' "וזה הוא ההפרש בין ט"ב ליוה"כ, דביוה"כ אין
לאכול רק במקום סכנה, ובט"ב אפילו שלא במקום סכנה, דבמקום חולי
לא גזרו רבנן ולכן כתב הטור בשם הרמב"ן וכן רבינו הב"י בסע' ו' דחיה כל
ל' יום, וכן חולה שהוא צריך לאכול א"צ אומד אלא מאכלין אותו מיד
דבמקום חולי לא גזרו רבנן עכ"ל. ואפילו הוא חולי שאינו מוטל במטה,
דאילו במוטל במטה גם ביה"כ כ' אינו מתענה דכל שמוטל במטה הוא בסכנה
כדמוכח בשבת דף לב, ע"ש. ויתבאר בסי' תרי"ח בס"ד, אבל בעלי מיחושים
בעלמא מתענים. כללו של דבר: כל שהוא בגדר חולה אינו מתענה בט"ב,
וכל שאינו בגדר חולה מתענה וסתם עוברות ומניקות מתענות אא"כ
חלושות וקרובות לחולי וכו' עכ"ל.

19. ועיין מה שכתבנו בפרק 17 הערה 35.

20. המשנה ברורה בסי' תקנ"ד בביאור הלכה ד"ה "דבמקום חולי" כתב שיש
ענין לאכול פחות פחות מכשיעור דבזה לא נעקר התענית לגמרי ורחמנא
ליבא בעי. אולם הערוך השולחן בסי' תקנ"ד סע' ז' כתב שבט' באב אין
ענין לאכול פחות מכשיעור כיון דט' באב הוא דרבנן. ועיין בשו"ת ציץ
אליעזר ח"י סי' כ"ה פרק ט"ו מה שכתב בזה.

21. עיין תורת היולדת פרק מ"ח הע' ה', ו'.

22. שו"ת ציץ אליעזר חלק י' סי' כ"ה פרק כ"ב.

23. לפי הוראת הגר"מ אליהו.

24. שו"ת יחוה דעת ח"ג סי' מ'.

25. כף החיים סי' תקנ"ו אות ט' ובשו"ת יחוה דעת שם.

26. שו"ע או"ח תקנ"ד סי' ה'.

פרק 8

1. רמב"ם הל' דעות פ"ד ה"א.

2. כמו שאומרים חז"ל, יפה שעה אחת בעולם הזה וכו'.

3. שבת קכ"ט, א' "רב ושמואל דאמרי תרוייהו כל המיקל בסעודת הקזת דם מקילין לו מזונותיו מן השמים ואומרים הוא על חייו לא חס אני אחוס עליו".

4. ויקרא רבה ל"ד, ג'.

5. רמב"ם הל' דעות שם הל' ט"ו.

6. משלי כ"א, כ"ג.

7. רמב"ם שם.

8. יומא מ"ז, א'.

9. שופטים פרק י"ג. ועיין בספר מוסר הנביאים שם (ולרב יהודה לייב גינצבורג, הוצאת פלדהיים).

10. כתובות ס', ב'. ועיין שם עוד דוגמאות נוספות.

11. עיין ביומא מ"ז, א', בסיפור על רבי ישמעאל בן קמחית (ולפי האיכא דאמרי), וידועים הדברים שגם מחשבות של הבעל והאשה בשעת הזיווג משפיעות ביצירת נפש הולד, ועיין בספר בעלי נפש להראב"ד בשער הקדושה.

12. רמב"ם הלכות דעות פ"ד הי"ג.

13. קיצור שולחן ערוך סי' ל"ב סע' ב'.

14. רמב"ם שם הל' ב', ו', י"א, י"ג, י"ד.

16. יומא ע"ה, ב'.

17. קיצור שלחן ערוך סי' ל"ב סע' י', וכן דעת רבי אליעזר בענין חובת אכילה בסוכה "תשבו כעין תדורו" י"ד סעודות (סוכה כ"ז, א'), ובעיקר נלמד מהאמור בשמות ט"ז, ח' "ויאמר משה בתת ה' לכם בערב בשר לאכל ולחם בבקר לשבע" (ואע"פ שבשבת אוכלין ג' סעודות, ביום ששי אוכלים רק סעודה אחת). וכן בקצש"ע שם.

18. שו"ע יו"ד סי' רנ"ג סע' א' הנוטלים מן התמחוי נוטלים ב' סעודות ביום, ועיין ט"ז שם.

19. מהרש"א יומא ע"ה ב': אהא דמשה רבינו קבע להם זמן סעודה "דהיינו זמן סעודה לכל אדם בשעת רביעית דהמן נלקט להם בבקר עד ג' שעות כדאמרינן פ' ת"ה ונמצא סעודה בשעה רביעית, וכן במס' שבת דף י', א' שעה רביעית מאכל מאכל כל אדם חמישית מאכל פועלים ששית מאכל ת"ח," וכן נפסק בשו"ע או"ח סי' קנ"ז "כשיגיע שעה רביעית יקבע סעודתו ואם הוא תלמיד חכם ועוסק בלימודו ימתין עד שעה ששית".

20. רמב"ם שם ה"ב.

21. רמב"ם שם ה"ו. בספר כף החיים סי' קנ"ז אות מ"ב כתב שפירות האילן שיש בהם טעם וריח כגון תפוחים ולימונים מתוקים גורמים טומאת קרי מאד.

23. רמב"ם שם ה"ז.
24. שמות ט"ז, ח'.
25. יומא ע"ה, ב'.
26. רש"י שם, וראה סימן קנ"ז משנה ברורה ס"ק ד' וכף החיים אות ל"ז ול"ח.
28. לדוגמא - דברי המחבר באו"ח סי' רצ"א סע' ה'.
29. וכן השפתי חכמים הסביר את רש"י. מופיע במהדורה המודפסת באוצר מפרשי רש"י.
30. רמב"ם שם ה"ה "ימתין שלוש או ארבע שעות".
31. וכן כתב המ"ב בסי' קנ"ז ס"ק ד' טוב שישים אכילתו. ביום קלה מבלילה.
32. עירובין נ"ה, ב'.
33. רש"י ורד"ק מלכים ב פרק ד' פסוק ל"ט.
34. ועיין כף החיים שם אות ל"ז ול"ח.
37. רמב"ם שם ה' כ"א.
38. מ"ב סי' קנ"ז ס"ק ד'.
54. קיצור שלחן ערוך סי' ל"ב סע' י"ז.
56. רמב"ם שם ה"ב וקצש"ע שם.
57. רמב"ם שם הל' י"ב.
58. קצש"ע שם.
59. קצש"ע שם סע' ט"ו.
60. בעלי הנפש להראב"ד פרק שער הקדושה הוצאת מוסד הרב קוק עמ' קכ"ה וקק"ו וז"ל "ושתי תקנות גדולות יש בענין הזה, האחת שלא תזיקנו אכילתו, והשנית כי היא כניעת היצר ושברון התאווה וכו'. ואין צריך לומר שישמור האדם את עצמו מן המאכלים שהוא מכיר שהן מזיקין אותו, כי האוכל מאכלים המזיקים אותו ואפשר לו זולתן הרי זה פושע בגופו ופושע בנפשו מפני שהוא הולך אחר תאוותו ואינו חושש על אבידת גופו והיא דרך היצה"ר ועצתו הסכלית להסיתו מדרך החיים אל דרך המות. וידע כל חי מדבר שאין דרך ליצה"ר עליו אלא מדרך ההיתר, ופתח דרכו מן המותר אצלו, ואם ישמור את הפתח אינו צריך שימור אחר".
61. רמב"ם שם הל' ט"ו.
62. רמב"ם שם ה"ב, והאוכל אכילה גסה ביום כיפור פטור, כיון שאינו נחשב אוכל.
63. קצש"ע שם סע' י'.
64. אורות התשובה, פרק א'.

פרק 9

1. רמב"ם הלכות דעות פ"ד ה' ב', ו' י"ג, י"ד.
4. רמב"ם שם ה"ד.

פרק 10

2. מתוך קונטרס "אחוותנו את היי לאלפי רבבה" (חיה אסתר ספקטור) עמוד 42-43.

קהלת רבה ז': "פועה זו מרים שהיתה פועה באשה והולד יוצא". ומסביר המתנות כהונה "מדברת ולחשה באזנה דבר מה והולד יוצא שלא בצער".

פרק 11

1. משנה שבת פרק ב' משנה ו'.
2. גמרא שם ל"ב, א'.
3. כתובות נ"ט, ב'.
4. עיין מלבי"ם ויקרא כ"ג, מ"ג ד"ה "כי בסכות הושבתי". ועיין בביאור הגר"א משלי א', א' שכתב שבכל דבר יש חומר ופועל וצורה ותכלית.

פרק 12

1. שו"ע או"ח סי' ש"ל ובמ"ב ס"ק א'.
2. הערות מהגר"מ שטרנבוך לספר תורת היולדת (ב).
3. ועיין שמירת שבת כהלכתה פרק מ' סעי' ס"ה. השיעור לתחום שבת הנ"ל הוא לפי הגר"ח נאה. לפי החזו"א 1160 מטר או 1269 ירד.
4. שהרי זה דומה לדין התיבה שיש בה דבר המותר בטלטול יחד עם דבר האסור בטלטול דאיתא בסי' ש"י סע' ט' דמותר לטלטל את התיבה, וכן הורה לי הגר"מ אליהו.
5. מכיון שהיא יוצאת בהיתר אין איסור להוציא חפצים אל מחוץ לתחום, וכך שמעתי מהגר"מ אליהו. ועיין שמירת שבת כהלכתה פרק מ' הע' קל"ו.
6. עיין מ"ב סי' ש"י סע' ל"ג ס"ק כ"ג ועי' שמירת שבת כהלכתה פרק מ' ס"ו. ועיין הלכות עירובין (רב לנגה) פרק ט' סעיף ט' ובהערה 225. ועיין תורת היולדת פרק ט"ז, וראה שמירת שבת כהלכתה פרק ל"א סע' ח' שפסק וז"ל ומותר לה לקחת עמה כל מה שהכרחי לה לשבת ולא תוכל להשיג בבית חולים אע"פ שאין עירוב במקום" עכ"ל. ועיין שו"ת מנחת יצחק חלק ח' סי' ל' בנוגע להבאת דברים ע"י נכרי, ועיין שו"ת ארץ צבי סי' ע"ה, בנוגע להבאת דברים ע"י קטן.
7. וכך הורה לי הגר"מ אליהו. ועיין תורת היולדת פרק י' שחולק.
8. שמירת שבת כהלכתה פרק ל"ב סע' מ' ותורת היולדת פ"ט אות א' מתירים ע"י שנים שעשאוה. ועיין בשמירת שבת כהלכתה שם שמתיר אף בהרמת השפופרת בשתי ידיים. ובשו"ת ציץ אליעזר חי"ז סי' כ' אות ג' נוטה לאסור ע"י שנים שעשאוה.
9. שמירת שבת כהלכתה פרק ל"ב סע' מ"א.
10. שו"ת ציץ אליעזר חי"ג סי' נ"ה.
11. עיין שו"ע או"ח סי' שכ"ח סע' י"ב ובהגה שם, ועיין שם בט"ז ס"ק ה' שפסק כמו המחבר, וכן פסק הא"ר שם ס"ק י"ב, וכן פסק הגרש"ז סע' י"ג, וכף החיים ס"ק ע"ד, ובערוך השולחן סע' ז'. ועיין בשו"ת ציץ אליעזר ח"ח סי' ט"ו פרק ב', וראה שמירת שבת כהלכתה פרק ל"ב הערה קי"א. וראה שו"ת אור לציון לגאון הרב בן ציון אבא שאול ח"ב עמ' רנ"ה אות ג'.
12. עיין תורת היולדת, פרק כ"ג. ועיין שמירת שבת כהלכתה פרק ל"ב סע' נ"ו.
13. שמירת שבת כהלכתה פרק ל"ו סע' ח'.
14. מ"ב סי' ש"ל ס"ק ט'.
15. הגמ' במסכת שבת קכ"ח, ב' מתירה להדליק נר בשביל היולדת ואפילו לסומא. מפני שמתישבת דעתה בזה, שהיא סבורה שאם יש משהו שיש לעשותו תראה חברתה ותעשה. מכאן אנו לומדים שמותר לחלל שבת עבור

היולדת, ולו רק כדי ליישב דעתה. הסיבה לכך היא שהפחד עלול להביא את היולדת למצב של סכנה.

וכך הוא גם בעניין נסיעה לבית החולים. אם מתישבת דעתה בכך שנמצא איתה מלווה שהיא סומכת עליו מותר ואף חייב לנסוע עמה בשבת. וכן כותב החזון איש בקובץ איגרות וז"ל: "בעניין נסיעת יולדת בשבת... מזרז אני שיסעו עמה". שו"ת אג"מ או"ח ח"א סי' קל"ב מחלק בין הדלקת נר (המוזכרת בגמרא) לבין נסיעה. כי בשעת הלידה דרך כל אדם לפחד שמא לא יראו מה נחוץ ליולדת דאף שהמילדת אומרת שבקיאה היא גם בלא נר ודאי רשאית היולדת שלא להאמין לה. אבל בעניין הנסיעה אל לה לפחד כי היא יודעת שאין שום צורך (אמיתי) ותועלת בנסיעת הבעל או האם איתה, ורק "תונבא בעלמא" הוא הפחד שלה לנסוע לבדה. ואולי פחד כזה אינו גדול כל כך שיביא לסכנה, כיוון שאין שום טעם לפחדה.

וכתב עוד שם וז"ל, אבל מכל מקום לדינא כיוון דמצינו ביולדת שעלולה להסתכן מחמת פחד מי הוא שיכול לסמוך על חילוקים בחשש פיקוח נפש. לכן אם אומרת שהיא מפחדת אף אחרי שמסבירין לה שאין לה ממה לפחד ליסע לבד יש בזה חשש פק"נ וצריכים הבעל או האם ליסע עמה. ואף אם נוסעת לבית החולים כשעדיין אינה צועקת בחבליה אם הוא במקום רחוק יש לו ג"כ ליסע עמה, דאף שעתה לא תסתכן היא, אבל הא אפשר שבאמצע הדרך יתוספו לה חבלי לידה עד השיעור שתצעק בחבליה שאז יש לחוש שמא תסתכן מחמת פחדה, עכ"ל האג"מ.

אע"פ שבתחילת התשובה חילק הרב פיינשטיין זצ"ל חילק בין הדלקת נר לנסיעה, בסוף התשובה היקל עד כדי היתר נסיעה עוד טרם התחזקות הצירים והפחד שתתפחד, מ"מ נראה שהוא מתיר רק במקרה שהאשה מבקשת אף אחרי שמסבירים לה שאין לה סיבה לפחד. ונראה לי שאפשר לצרף עוד נימוק להתיר: כי בזמן שנכתבה התשובה הזאת באג"מ, לא היה נהוג כ"כ שהבעל או האם ישארו עמה בחדר לידה. אבל בזמננו מקובל מאוד הדבר שהבעל ישאר בחדר לידה לפחות עד הלידה כדי ליישב דעתה. (עיין לקמן פרק 13) ואם הוא לא יסע עמה, גם לא יוכל להיות עמה בחדר לידה כדי ליישב דעתה, וא"כ ודאי מותר לו ליסע עימה לביה"ח, כדי שבחדר הלידה יוכל ג להיות עמה וליישב דעתה. אולם לאלו שלא נהגו שהבעל יהיה עמה בחדר לידה נראה שאין טעם להתיר אלא א"כ היא מפחדת בעת הנסיעה. ואמנם פעמים רבות אם ילדים מעדיפה שהבעל ישאר עם הילדים בבית, והיא תסתדר לבדה בנסיעה. לכן צריך לברר אצל כל אשה שמא היא רק מתפנקת ואילו היה צורך בהשארתו בבית היתה אומרת לבעלה שלא לבוא עמה.

16. שמירת שבת כהלכתה פרק מ', סע' נ"ז.
17. שם פרק מ' סע' נ"ט, ס'.
18. עיין שו"ת אג"מ ח"ד סי' פ', ועיין בשו"ת מנחת שלמה סי' ח', ושמירת שבת כהלכתה פרק ל"ו סי' ה'

פרק 13

2. וכן הורו לי הגר"מ אליהו והגרח"פ שיינברג. ואע"פ שבשו"ת אג"מ יו"ד ח"ד סי' ע"ו כתב שאין מציאות כזאת. היום אנו יודעים שקיימת מציאות כזאת, ואולי אפשר להתירה על פי דברי החזו"א ביו"ד סי' פ"ג אות א' וז"ל

"דשמעינן דפתיחת הקבר דבגמרא הוא אתערותא דלידה" עכ"ל. וכיון
שהפתיחה הזאת היא פתיחה פיזיולוגית ולא מחמת הלידה אין לטמאה. וגם
אפשר לצרף את דעת החוו"ד דפה"ק בלא דם הוא דוקא כשיצא דבר
מהקבר כמו ולד, לכן אין לטמאה בפתיחה פיזיולוגית.

3. בספר בדי השלחן סי' קצ"ד ס"ק ל' כתב בשם בעלי הוראה שדינה כנדה.
גם בספר שיעורי שבט הלוי, עמוד רמ"ט, כתב נראה להחמיר כשהמצב הוא
ממש לפני הלידה, שיש לחוש שדם עם המים. ובספר תורת היולדת פרק
י"ח סע' ה' כתב וז"ל "ירדו המים, מורים בעלי הוראה שלא יגע בה בעלה
כדין נדה, אלא א"כ הוא צורך גדול ואין אחר שיעזור לה". ובהערה ו' כתב
"דאין צריך לחשוש שמעורב דם במים. ויש המחלקים בין ירידת קצת מים
לירידת כל המים בפעם אחת שאז פי השליא פתוח ויש לחוש שמעורב בו
דם". ובספר מחשבת הטהרה פרק י"א הערה 2, כתב בשם הגאון רבי שלמה
זלמן אויערבך להתיר בזה. ומכל מקום נכון לברר אם לא נתערב דם במים
ואז היא טהורה ללא כל חשש. אבל כבר כתבנו שאסור לבדוק לצורך זה כי
הבדיקה עלולה לגרום זיהום חלילה. ובספר טהרת הבית (חלק ב' עמוד נ"ג)
פסק הגאון הרב עובדיה יוסף וז"ל "כל שאין רואים דם עם המים אין לחוש
לכולם דאחזוקי איסורא לא מחזיקינן." אולם שמעתי מהגר"מ אליהו שיש
להחמיר, וכן שמעתי מהגרח"פ שיינברג.

4. דקי"ל אין פתיחת הקבר בלא דם (יו"ד סי' קצ"ד סע' ב') ואומרת הגמרא
בשבת קכ"ט א': "מאימתי פתיחת הקבר? אמר אביי משעה שתשב על
המשבר רב הונא בריה דרב יהושע אמר משעה שהדם שותת ויורד, ואמרי
לה משעה שחברותיה נושאות אותה באגפיה" וכתב הסדרי טהרה סי' קצ"ד
אות כ"ה "ומ"ש בספר כו"פ דבאותה שעה צריך הבעל להזהר בה נ"ל דלאו
דוקא באותה שעה שישבה על המשבר אלא מיד שאחזוה צירים וחבלי לידה
ומבקשת להביא לה חכמה על המשבר צריך הבעל להזהר בה דודאי לאו ישיבת המשבר
גורם פה"ק אלא כל שהיא קרובה ללידה כ"כ שצריכה לישב על המשבר
ואיכא למיחש אלו היתה היתה המילדת מזומנת אצלה היתה מושיבה מיד על
המשבר לכן צריך להיות נזהר בה" עכ"ל. וכן פסק בשו"ת אג"מ יו"ד ח"ד
סי' ע"ה.

5. על פי דברי הרמ"א ביו"ד סי' קצ"ה סע' ז' וי"ז.

6. כתב הסדרי טהרה ביו"ד סי' קצ"ד ס"ק כ"ה ובשו"ת נחלת שבעה סי' ט'
באשה שמלאו ימיה ללדת לפי דמיונה וקראו למילדת וגם שאר נשים
הסכימו שהגיע עתה עת ללדת והתעסקו עמה ואחר איזה שעות המילדת לא
ראתה את הוולד ועדיין היא הולכת כמו ד' שבועות אח"ז וכריסה בין
שיניה, והנשים מעידות שבכל מדינות פולין המנהג שתיכף שקראו למילדת
והיא בודקת את האשה אם הגיע זמנה ללדת או לאו מחזיקינן אותה
בטומאה, והאריך לעשות סמוכות למנהג ע"פ הדין מהא דאיתא בפרק
מפנין דפתיחת הקבר הוא משתמש על המשבר, והא קיי"ל דא"א לפתיחת
בקבר בלא דם, לכן טמאה משישבה על המשבר. וכ' ע"ז בס' סולת למנחה
וז"ל ולענ"ד אין דבריו ברורים וכ"ש אין מוכרחים דאף דקיי"ל דמשתשב
על המשבר הוי פה"ק, היינו כ"כ יולדת אח"כ מתוך קישוי זה משא"כ אם
אינה יולדת אח"כ, והלכה זמן רב ולא ילדה איגלאי מילתא למפרע שטעות
היה וחבלי שוא היה היה גם המילדת טעתה. וראיה ברורה לזה שכן איתא בפ"ז

דאהלות מ"ד דמשנפתח הקבר אין פנאי להלך ועיין בתוי"ט, וא"כ זו שהלכה
אח"כ מוכח שלא היה פה"ק,
גם נ"ל דבכה"ג לא שייך מנהג כי הוא דבר שאינו מצוי שתטעה המילדת וכל
הנשים ושתלך האשה אחר ישיבתה על המשבר כמה ימים ובדבר שאינו
מצוי לא שייך מנהג, ולענין שבת דמחללין ביושבת על המשבר משום
דאזלינן בתר רוב נשים וחזקת המילדות הבקיאות שיודעין זמן הלידה וכו'
גם לא יהא אלא ספק הא קיי"ל ספק פק"נ מחללין השבת עכ"ל ובספר כו"פ
מסיק דבאותה שעה באמת יש לבעל להזהר בה אבל כאשר ראינו שפסקו
הצירים ועמדה מן המשבר ולא ילדה איתגלי מילתא דלא כן היה וכאב
בעלמא הוא דכאיב לה ולא היה מעיקרא פה"ק דלא שכיח שיהיה נפתח
ויחזור ויסתום חבלי לידה, לכן נראה שלא היה פה"ק וטהורה וכן המנהג
בכל מקום, מיהו במקום דנהגו איסור יש להניח מנהגן כי הוא חומרא שיש
בו קצת טעם ומקום לסמוך ע"כ דבריו".
ואע"פ שהסדרי טהרה תמה על הסולת למנחה במה שהביא ראיה מהמשנה
באהלות ע"ש מ"מ מסכים לדבריו דאתגלי למפרע שהיא טעתה וסברה
שהם חבלי לידה ובאמת טהורה היא כיון שלא שכיח שיחזור ויסתם לאחר
שנפתח. וע"ש שהסיק שיש שתי פתיחות: יש פתיחה שיטמא הולד המת
באהל ולא יחשב בלוע ובזה צריך פה"ק בשעור רב דהיינו כראש פיקה. ויש
פתיחה שמתירה לחלל שבת בעבורה ולחשבה לנדה וזה הוי אפילו פתיחה
מועטת.
ובעצם עיקר הדין דפה"ק יש מחלוקת. לדעת הראב"ד רמב"ן ורשב"א אין
פה"ק בלא דם, אבל הרמב"ם בהלכות איסורי ביאה פ"ה הל' י"ג פסק
דאפשר פה"ק בלא דם, ועיין במגיד משנה שבירר את הסוגיא. וגם אם
נאמר דאין פה"ק בלא דם, לפה"ק דהא הכוונה היא שמעת שיצא
מהרחם דבר א"א מבלי שיצא דם בהכרח, וכן פסק החוות דעת וז"ל "דהא
דאמרינן דא"א לפתיחת הקבר בלא דם היינו דוקא כשהפילה איזה דבר
דנפתח הקבר כ"כ עד שיצא ממנה אז אמרינן דא"א בלא דם, אבל כשנפתח
הקבר ולא יצא ממנה אף דם אינו יוצא" עכ"ל וכן פסק הגאון הרב ברוך
פרנקל זצ"ל בהגהותיו על הנודע ביהודה סימן ק"כ. ובספר תשובה מאהבה
בסי' קט"ז כתב וז"ל הנה כבר סיבר עמי בזה הגאון רבי מאיר פישלס זצ"ל
והורתי להקל ומה לנו בדברי קצת ליקוטים המתפשטים למצוא חומרות
חדשות. ואמנם בעל נחלת שבעה מחמיר בזה אך אין להשגיח על חלומותיו
ועל דבריו בזה, דמה בכך אם הוא התחלת פתיחת הקבר הרי רז"ל שאמרו
א"א לפה"ק בלא דם היינו כשיצא מהרחם דבר גוש כמו ולד או חתיכה כל
שאינה דקה כשפופרת דקה של קש אמרינן בודאי שיצא דם עמה אבל על
פתיחת הקבר לבד ולא יצא ממנה גוש לא אמרו שא"א בלא דם וכו', ומכל
שכן שעצם הדין שא"א לפה"ק בלא דם אינו מוסכם והרמב"ם פסק להקל
ואף דאנן קייומא לן לחומרא כמבואר בשו"ע קפ"ח סע' ג', היינו על כל פנים
בהרגישה בפתיחת הקבר שאז הוא ספק איסור כרת וכו' וכיון שאין כאן
איסור תורה וגם יש כאן ספק ספקא להקל שמא אין זה נחשב פתיחת הקבר
ושמא הלכה כהרמב"ם" עכ"ל.
וכמעט כל הפוסקים דחו את דברי הנחלת שבעה להלכה והם החת"ס ביו"ד
סי' קע"ט, הבית מאיר דף ס"ה, הערוך השולחן בסי' קצ"ד סע' נ"ג ועיין עוד

בספר טהרת הבית ח"ב במשמרת הטהרה דף נ' מהגאון הרב עובדיה יוסף
שהביא הרבה פוסקים שפסקו כסולת למנחה וכו"פ וסד"ט להתירה
לבעלה.

ובשו"ת אג"מ יו"ד ח"ב סי' ע"ו דן בשאלה האם היא חייבת לעשות בדיקה
לכל הפחות, וכתב שזה תלוי במחלוקת הסדרי טהרה והחוות דעת, שלדעת
הסדרי טהרה כיון דאיגלאי שלא היתה פה"ק אין צריך בדיקה כלל. ולדעת
החוות דעת אפשר דיש פתיחה רק שאין זו פתיחה דאמרינן את הכלל שאין
פה"ק בלא דם, תצטרך לעשות בדיקה, כי אין לומר בודאי לא יצא דם, דהא
גם לא נמצא בגמרא שלכן מסתברא שהוא ספק שמא יצא דם ותועיל
בדיקה. וכתב האג"מ שם "משמע שרוב האחרונים סברי דאיגלאי שהיה
טעות ולא נפתח הקבר כלל וכן הוא בחת"ס חיו"ד סי' קע"ט דלכן אין
להצריך בדיקה אך אולי מהראוי להחמיר לכתחלה לחוש להחו"ד להצריכה
לבדוק אבל כשלא עשתה בדיקה שהוא לאסור אין להחמיר כלל" עכ"ל,
והגר"ע יוסף כתב על דברים אלו במשמרת הטהרה אינו מוכרח שאף
לכתחלה נראה שאינה צריכה בדיקה, והרי היא בחזקת טהורה. וכן משמעות
האחרונים להקל אף בלא בדיקה. ומ"מ המחמירה על עצמה לבדוק תבוא
עליה ברכה" עכ"ל.

ונראה דהלכה למעשה יש להתחשב במציאות הרפואית המודרנית. כי נקודת
המחלוקת בין הנחלת שבעה והסדרי טהרה וסיעתו היא, האם אמרינן
שהיתה פתיחה או לאו. לפי הנ"ש אמרינן שהיתה פתיחה ולפי הסד"ט
וסיעתו אמרינן שאיגלאי שלא היתה פתיחה. במציאות המעשית היום
אפשר לעשות בדיקה פשוטה כדי לברר אם אכן היתה פתיחה או לא. אם
היתה פתיחה אפילו מועטת (כפסק הסד"ט וכתב האג"מ שם שלדינא צריך
להחמיר כמוהו), היא אסורה לבעלה עד שתספור ז' נקיים.. ואם אין פתיחה
מותרת לבעלה (ובודאי אפשר להאמין למילדת או לרופא אפילו גוי, כיון
שבודקים לצורך הטיפול בה ויהיה לו גדר של מסיח לפי תומו יהיה נאמן
מכח שאומו לא מירע אומנותיה). לכן נראה שאין לקבוע יתדות בזה, אלא
נלך אחר המציאות: אם יש פתיחה ולו במעט טמאה וצריכה ז' נקיים ואם
לאו טהורה היא. ואולם בשעת הצורך כגון שהצירים היו זמן רב קודם
תאריך הלידה המשוער אולי נוכל לסמוך על דעת החוו"ד שאינה נטמאת
כשלא יצא דבר (שלכתחלה פסק האג"מ וכן הורה לי הגר"מ אליהו שיש
להחמיר כסד"ט) ולהתירה לבעלה. ויש לשאול מורה הוראה.

7. כפי שכבר בארנו מהרגע שיש צירים אמיתיים היא נחשבת נדה ובודאי
כשהיא יושבת על המשבר (המטה המיוחדת) היא נחשבת לנדה.

8. שו"ע יו"ד סי' קצ"ה סע' ז' "לא יסתכל אפילו בעקבה ולא במקומות
המכוסים שבה". ובאו"ח סי' ר"מ סע' ד'.

9. שו"ת מנחת יצחק ח"ח סי' ל'. וגם הוא התיר בצורך גדול ועיין בספר דרכי
טהרה דף קי"א שכתב "בשעת הלידה ולפניה אין לבעל לנגוע באשתו או
להסתכל בה במקומות המכוסים, אלא יעודדנה בדברים מפתח חדר
הלידה. והתבוננות זו אסורה יש בה כדי להרחיק את האהבה מביניהם
ולגנותה בעיניו."

10. שו"ת אג"מ יו"ד ח"ב סי' ע"א וז"ל "ובאם הבעל יכול להיות שמה להשגיח
שתעשה הדבר בסדר הנכון וגם לחזק אותה ולאמץ לבה, הנה אם יש צורך
אינו רואה איסור ואף בלא צורך איני רואה איסור, אבל אסור לו להסתכל

ביציאת הולד ממש שהרי אסור להסתכל במקומות המכוסים שבה בנדתה
ובמקום התורפה הוא אסור אפילו בטהורה, אך כשיזהר שלא להסתכל
ליכא איסור, וע"י מראה נמי אסור לבעל להסתכל" עכ"ל. הנה מפורש
בדבריו שמותר לבעל להיות נוכח בשעת הלידה אף ללא צורך, ולא כמו
שכתבו כמה מהמלקטים שלדעת הגר"מ פיינשטיין מותר לבעל להיות בחדר
לידה רק כשהאשה נפחדת או רק באופן שיש צורך.

וכן פסק הגר"ע יוסף בטהרת הבית ח"ב עמ' קס"ו וז"ל "מותר לבעל להיות
נוכח בחדר לידה בשעה שאשתו יולדת, כדי להשגיח שהכל יעשה בסדר
נכון, וגם כדי לחזק את רוחה ולאמץ את לבבה. ומכל שכן כשרואה שהיא
רגישה מאד ונתקפת אימה ופחדים בשעה שאוחזים אותה צירים וחבלי
לידה, שאז נוכחותו נחוצה ביותר. אולם אסור לו להסתכל בה בשעת יציאת
הולד, אלא יהפוך פניו לצד אחר" עכ"ל, ובהערה כ"ח כתב שהפסק של
המנחת יצחק נראה כחומרא יתירה לגדר.

11. ראה מאמרו של הרב יהודה הרצל הנקין אסיא י"ט שנת תשל"ח, ובספר
אסיא ב' עמ' 117 בתגובה של הרב משה הלברשטאם שליט"א שם, ועיין
בספר אסיא חלק ו' שהשיב על טענותיו.

12. על פי דברי הרמ"א ביו"ד סי' קצ"ה סע' ט"ז וי"ז. ועיין בתורת היולדת
פרק ל"א הערות ג' ד' וה'. ולכאורה גם אפשר לצרף את דעת החוו"ד בסי'
קצ"ד שהיולדת אינה נחשבת לנדה עד שיצא משהו מהמחבר כמו שכבר
בארנו. ועיין בספר בדי השולחן סי' קצ"ד ביאורים ד"ה מפני שא"א לפה"ק
בלא דם, ובטהרת הבית ח"ב במשמרת הטהרה אות כ"ח.

13. שו"ע או"ח סי' ד' סע' י"ט מ"ב ס"ק מ"ו.

14. שו"ע או"ח סי' רכ"ג סע' א' ומ"ב ס"ק ב' וס"ק ז' ועיין בביאור הלכה
שם. ובערוך השולחן שם סע' א' כתב שאין מברכין כלל על לידת הבת ועיין
במרומי שדה לנצי"ב ברכות נ"ד ד"ה "והנה", שלדעתו יש לברך על לידת בת
ועיין שם טעמו. וסיים "ואינבא לא ראיתי זאת בפוסקים ואולי יש לומר
וכו'" עיין שם. ועיין בשו"ת ציץ אליעזר חי"ג סי' כ' שכתב שיש לברך
שהחיינו על לידת בת כמו שפסק במשנה ברורה. ועיין בתשובות והנהגות
הרב משה שטרנבוך חלק ב' סי' קל"ג.

15. בענין ברכת הטוב והמטיב כתב המחבר בסי' רכ"ג סי' א' בהדיא שגם
האשה צריכה לברך. ועיין בשו"ת ציץ אליעזר חי"ד סי' כ"ב שפסק שבזמננו
גם האשה מברכת על לידת בת שהחיינו.

16. מ"ב שם ס"ק א' וס"ק ג', וראה כף החיים אות ה' וסי' ש"ל ה"ד "אם
עדיין תוקף השמחה בלבו אבל אח"כ יברך בלא שם ומלכות" עכ"ל. אם
האב לא היה נוכח בשעת הלידה ונולד לו בן מברך הטוב ומטיב כשיקבל
את הבשורה. ואם נולדה לו בת עיין במ"ב ס"ק ב' שדוקא כשרואה אותה
מברך שהחיינו. אבל לפי מה שכתב השו"ת ציץ אליעזר בחלק י"ד סי' כ"ב
שבזמנינו יש יותר שמחה בלידת בת מבזמנה, יתכן כמו בלידת בן, שיש
לברך מיד כשישמע וצ"ע.

17. בן איש חי פרשת ראה ש"א אות ח' עיין שם, וכף החיים רכ"ג אות ו'
וראה בילקוט יוסף ח"ג רכ"ג סי' ה'.

פרק 14

9. שו"ת אג"מ יו"ד ח"ב סי' ע"ד. וטעמו העיקרי הוא משום "דלידה בזמנה

כדרך הנשים לא נחשב לסכנה כלל, דמאחר שכן ברא השי"ת את העולם
שיפרו וירבו ובודאי ברא שיהיה לברכה ולא לסכנה, וגם הא ציוה השי"ת
בחיוב עשה להוליד בנים ולא מסתבר שיהיה הציווי ליכנס בסכנה בשביל
קיום עשה זו דפו"ר, ובפרט שהנשים אין מחוייבות בהעשה דפו"ר שנצטרך
לומר שנתנה התורה להם רשות ליכנס בסכנה להוליד בנים, אלא צ"ל שאין
בזה סכנה כלל, היינו שהבטיח השי"ת שלא יהיה בזה סכנה לעולם וכו', אבל
כשרוצין להקדים הלידה שלא כפי שהיה צריך להיות ליכא על זה הבטחתו,
וממילא נכנסה לסכנה דלידה שלולא הבטחת השי"ת הרי זה סכנה, ולכן הוא
דבר אסור לעשות תחבולות להקדים לידה, אם לא כשאיכא סכנה
לחכות."

10. טהרת הבית ח"ב עמ' נ"ד.

11. האפריון בספר בראשית, מובא בתורת היולדת פרק א' הערה א' עיין
שם. וגם כתב בשם הגרי"ש אלישיב שליט"א שמאחר ונאמר במשנה
באבות פ"ד כ"ב "על כרחך אתה נוצר וע"כ אתה נולד" יש להשאיר את שעת
הלידה לבורא עולם.

12. נדה ל, ב.

13. עיין פתחי תשובה יו"ד סי' קצ"ד ס"ק ד' ועיין שו"ת אג"מ או"ח ח"ג סי'
ק'.

פרק 15

1. על פי שו"ע או"ח סי' רס"ג סע' ו' ועיין היטב בביה"ל ד"ה בחורים.

2. שם מ"ב ס"ק ב'. וראה שמירת שבת כהלכתה ח"ב פרק מ"ה סע' ו'.

3. עיין בשו"ת יחוה דעת ח"ה סי' כ"ד. ובספר תורת היולדת כתב שאין לברך
על תאורה פלואורסנטית.

4. שם סע' ח' לדעת המחבר.

5. שם לדעת הרמ"א.

6. שם.

7. שם ועיין בשמירת שבת כהלכתה שם הערה ל"ב.

8. שם.

9. שם מ"ב ס"ק ל"ח.

10. ראה מ"ב שם ס"ק י"א שכתב שהמנהג שהבעל מדליק. והגר"ב פרנקל
כתב שהטעם שהבעל מדליק כי היולדת אינה זהה ממקומה. הערוך השולחן
כתב דוקא משום שהיא אינה נקיה מדם, אבל היום נוהגים שאשה שאינה
נקיה מדם מדליקה ומברכת, והיום נשים קמות מהמטה, לכן המנהג היום
שהאשה תדליק. ועיין בספר אוצר 'הברית של הרב יוסף דוד ויסברג פרק
ה'.

11. אוצר הברית פרק ה' סע' ב'.

12. שו"ע או"ח סי' רע"ג סע' א.

13. שו"ע או"ח סי' רע"ב סע' ט'. ועיין בשמירת שבת כהלכתה ח"ב פרק נ"ג
סע' ט"ו.

14. שו"ת משיב דבר ח"א סי' כ"א, ש"ש כהלכתה ח"ב פרק נ"ה סע' י"ז.

15. ראה הלכות צבא (הרב זכריה בן שלמה עמוד 115).

16. או"ח סי' רפ"ט ובמ"ב סק"י.

17. או"ח סי' רפ"ט סע' ב.

18. אג"מ או"ח ח"ב סי' ע"ה.
19. שו"תאג"מ שם. שו"ת ציץ אליעזר ח"ח סי' ט"ז. וכן בערוך השולחן רצ"ו סע' י"ג.
20. שו"ת יחוה דעת ח"ב סי' ל"ח.
21. שמירת שבת כהלכתה ח"ב פרק ס' סע' ה'.
22. ערוך השולחן שם, ואג"מ שם.
23. שו"ע או"ח סי' רצ"ו סע' ח' ומ"ב שם.
ולגבי נשים בברכת הנר עיין בביה"ל סי' רצ"ד ד"ה "לא יבדילו" שהסתפק אם נשים מברכות על הנר והכריע דיותר נכון לומר דאינו חייבת בברכת הנר לכו"ע. ופסק האג"מ בחושן משפט ח"ב סי' מ"ז אות ב' שמברכות על הנר וכך פסק בילקוט יוסף ח"ד סי' רצ"ו סע' י"ג. בשמירת שבת כהלכתה ח"ב פרק ס"א סע' כ"ד כתב שטוב לסדר ברכת הנר אחר שתייה מהכוס שלא יהיה חשש להפסק. אולם באג"מ הנ"ל לא הזכיר חילוק זה.
24. שו"ע או"ח סי' רצ"ו מ"ב ס"ק ל"ה. ילקוט יוסף ח"ד סי' רצ"ו סע' י"ג.
25. שם סי' רצ"ז סע' א', ועיין מ"ב שם טעם הדבר.
26. שם סי' רח"צ סע' א'.
27. שם סע' ב' ומ"ב שם.
28. שו"ע או"ח סי' רצ"ו מ"ב ס"ק ל"ו.
29. שו"ת אג"מ או"ח ח"ד סי' צ"א אות ד'.
30. מ"ב סי' רס"ב ס"ק ה'.

פרק 16

1. ויקרא י"ב א', ה'.
2. עמוד האמת פרשת תזריע.
3. נצי"ב העמק הדבר ריש פרשת תזריע.
4. ברכות ל"א, א'.
5. שו"ע יו"ד סי' קצ"ד סע' א'. ודין יוצא דופן: אם לא יצא דם אלא דרך דופן אמו טהורה מלידה ומנדה ומזיבה. (שם סי' י"ד). אבל מציאות כזאת אינה שכיחה.

פרק 17

1. שו"ע או"ח סי' ש"ל סע' ד'.
2. מ"ב שם ס"ק י"ג .
3. מ"ב שם סוף ס"ק י"ד "דלב יודע מרת נפשו".
4. עיין שמירת שבת כהלכתה פרק ל"ב סע' פ"ג ובתורת היולדת פרק ל"ה.
5. ועיין בשמירת שבת כהלכתה פרק ל"ב הערה ר"כ.
6. שו"ע או"ח סי' ש"ל סע' ד'.
7. ראה שמירת שבת כהלכתבה פרק ל"ו סע' י"ד.
8. שו"ע שם ומ"ב ס"ק ט"ו וט"ז.
9. שמירת שבת כהלכתה פרק ל"ו סי' ט"ו ועיין שם בפרק ל"ג סע' ב'.
10. מ"ב שם ס"ק ט"ו, ובשער הציון אות י"ג בשם פמ"ג, ובשמירת שבת כהלכתה פרק ל"ו סע' ט"ו.
11. שו"ע או"ח סי' תרי"ז סע' ד'.
12. כך משמע מן השו"ע בסי' תרי"ח סע' א'.

13. מ"ב סי' תרי"ז ס"ק י', ושער הציון אות י"ב וכן בבבה"ל סי' תרי"ח ד"ה "כשמאכלין" בשם הגרב"פ.

14. שו"ע הרב בעל התניא סי' תרי"ז סע' ד' וסי' תרי"ח סע' י"ג. והובאה דעתו במ"ב הנ"ל וכן בבבה"ל הנ"ל וכן פסק הכף החיים בסי' תרי"ז אות י"ט בשם מט"א, וגם כתב שכן משמע מסתימת השו"ע סי' תרי"ח סע' ז' וכן נפסק בשו"ת יחוה דעת ח"ו סי' ל"ט בהערה שם. ועיין בתורת היולדת פרק נ"א בהערות ד' וה' ובשו"ת יחוה דעת שם, שהאריכו לברר את הסוגיא. ועיין בשו"ת ציץ אליעזר חט"ו סי' י"ג

15. שמירת שבת כהלכתה פרק ל"ט הע' מ"ב בשם הגרש"ז אויערבך.

16. מ"ב סי' תרי"ז ס"ק י' ובבה"ל סי' תרי"ח ד"ה כשמאכלין, על פי המגן אברהם סי' תקי"ז ס"ק ג' וא"ר אות ב' מפקפק בזה.

17. ראה מאמרו של הרב חיים דוד הלוי בתחומין ח"ד עמ' 451 שהתיר לה לצום, אולם בסוף התשובה תלה את היתרו בהסכמת גדולי הוראה בדורנו. וראה ספר תורת היולדת פרק נ"א הע' י"ב, וראה שו"ת יחוה דעת חלק ו' סי' ל"ט שמשמע שאסור לה להתענות, וצ"ע לדינא.

18. שו"ע או"ח תרי"ז, מ"ב ס"ק י"א וכף החיים אות כ' ושו"ע הרב סע' ד'.

19. כף החיים שם. ושמירת שבת כהלכתה פ' ל"ט סע' י"ג.

20. מ"ב שם ושער הציון אות ט"ז.

21. כך משמע מן השו"ע ומן המ"ב שם. וכן בשמירת שבת כהלכתה פר' ל"ט סע' י"ג.

22. שו"ע או"ח סי' תרי"ז סע' ד' ומ"ב שם ס"ק י"ב על פי א"ר אות ג'.

23. עיין בכף החיים סי' תקנ"ד אות כ"ח. 24. ועיין בשו"ת יחוה דעת חלק א' סימן ס"א. וכן פסק המ"ב בסי' תרי"ח ס"ק ה'

25. שו"ע או"ח סי' תרי"ב סע' א'. ומ"ב סי' תרי"ח ס"ק כ"א על פי תשו' חתם סופר. וראה שמירת שבת כהלכתה פרק ל"ט סע' י"ח והע' ע"א.

26. שו"ע או"ח סי' תרי"ב סע' ט' ומ"ב שם ס"ק ל"א. וסי' תרי"ח סע' ז'. וראה שמירת שבת כהלכתה פרק ל"ט סע' כ', תורת היולדת פרק נ"ב עמוד רנ"ו.

27. ספר החינוך מצוה שי"ג. שו"ת יחוה דעת ח"א סי' ט"ז. שמירת שבת כהלכתה פרק ל"ט סע' י"ט.

28. שמירת שבת כהלכתה פרק ל"ט סע' י"ח.

29. שמירת שבת כהלכתה שם סע' כ"א.

30. כל הנ"ל מלוקט בשמירת שבת כהלכתה פרק ל"ט סע' ל"א ובתורת היולדת פרק נ"ב סע' י"א - י"ד. עיין שם למקורות.

31. גם דינים אלו מלוקטים בשמירת שבת כהלכתה שם ובתורת היולדת שם.

32. עיין ט"ז סי' תקנ"ד ס"ק ה' שאסורה להתענות בשלשה ימים ראשונים. וא"ר כתב שאין לה להחמיר על עצמה תוך ז' ימים. עיין שם אות ח' ועיין בכף החיים סי' תקנ"ד אות ל"ו.

33. שו"ע או"ח סי' תקנ"ד סע' ו'.

34. שם. בהג"ה ומ"ב ס"ק י"ב. וכן דעת המהרש"ל (תשובות נ"ג) שיולדת תוך שלושים יום חייבת להתענות.

35. מ"ב שם בשם ליקוטי פר"ח וז"ל "דמסתמא מאכילין אותה". וכתב הערוך השולחן בסי' תקנ"ד סע' ח' שמה שכתב הרמ"א שנוהגות להתענות כל זמן שאין להן צער גדול "אולי זהו בימיהם שהדורות היו בריאים וחזקים

אבל עכשיו חלילה להיולדת להתענות בט"ב תוך שלשים כי עדיין חלושה
היא והיא ממש כחולה ולכן אין להניחן להתענות בט"ב. ועיין בכף החיים
אות כ"ט שהביא מתשובות המהר"ם מרוטנברג ד"בדורות חלושות הללו
ובפרט מי שיש לו מיחוש בחלל הגוף אין להחמיר בשום אופן וכך אני
מורה". וכן נפסק בשו"ת יחוה דעת ח"א סי' מ"ב ולדעתו אין לה להתענות
אפילו שעות. וכן בשו"ת ציץ אליעזר ח"י ס' כ"ה פרק ט"ז.

36. הלכה זו טעונה בירור. הטור בשם הרמב"ן כתב שרבנן לא גזרו על
החולה להתענות בט"ב, א"כ אין לחולה או ליולדת תוך ל' יום (שנחשבת
כחולה) מצוה להתענות כלל. לכאורה כיון שאינה מצווה להתענות אינה
צריכה גם להתענות אפילו כמה שעות, כיון שהצום אינו שייך לה כלל. וכן
פסק המחבר בסי' תקנ"ד סע' ו' וז"ל "חיה כל שלשים יום וכן חולה שהוא
צריך לאכול אין צריך אומר אלא מאכילין אותו מיד דבמקום חולי לא
גזרו רבנן". והנה בהלכות מילה יו"ד סי' רס"ה סע' ד' בענין שתיית הכוס
בברית מילה ביום צום כתב וז"ל" ביוה"כ ובד' צומות לא יברך על הכוס,
מיהו בג' צומות מהם שהיולדת אינה מתענה יכול לברך על הכוס ותטעום
ממנו היולדת וכו' אבל ביום הכיפורים וט"ב שאין היולדת יכולה לשתות
אין מברכין על הכוס" ע"כ.

לכאורה המחבר ביו"ד סותר את דבריו באו"ח, שבאו"ח כתב שחיה תוך ל'
יום מאכילין אותה מיד, ואילו ביו"ד משמע שהיא צריכה להתענות. סתירה
בולטת יותר נמצאת בין דבריו ביו"ד לדבריו ביו"ד סי' תקנ"ט סע' ז' ששם
כתב בפירוש "ואם היולדת נמצאת במקום המילה יברך על הכוס ותשתה
ממנו היולדת."

הבית הלל ביו"ד עמד על סתירה זו ותירץ שלמרות שבט"ב היא פטורה
מלהתענות, מכל מקום היא צריכה להתענות כמה שעות. ומיירי שהברית
בבוקר ולכן עדיין אינה יכולה לטעום. וקשה על תירוצו שהרי המנהג הוא
שעושים ברית מילה בט"ב אחר חצות או לפחות אחר אמירת קינות (סי'
תקנ"ט סע' ז') ועד אז בודאי היא יכולה לאכול ולשתות. ותו קשה, איזה
ענין יש לצום כמה שעות שהרי תענית שעות היא משום חינוך למצוות חינוך
אינה שייכת לגביה. ולפי רוב הדעות אפילו קטנים אינם שייכים במצות
חינוך של תענית שעות בט"ב. (ועיין בתורת היולדת פרק מ"ח סע' ה' שעמד
על השאלות הנ"ל.)

בשעה"צ סי' תקנ"ד סק"ב בשם הפר"ח תירץ שבסי' תקנ"ד ותקנ"ט מדובר
באשה רגילה שאינה חזקה במיוחד ואינה יכולה לצום, ומותר לה לאכול
ולשתות מיד, ואילו ביו"ד מדובר באשה חזקה ביותר שמסוגלת לסבול את
הצום ואסורה לאכול.

לפי חילוק זה אשה רגילה שאיננה צריכה לצום גם איננה צריכה לצום
תענית שעות, כיון שהיא בגדר של חולה וחז"ל לא גזרו על החולה, כמו
שפסק האבני נזר באו"ח סי' תקל"מ. מ"מ האו"ר והמ"ב בס"ק י"ד הביאו את
דברי בית הלל להלכה, שעליה לצום כמה שעות אם כן לא קשה לה.

גם החת"ס בתשובות או"ח סי' קנ"ז כתב אדות חולה האוכל בט' באב וז"ל
"לא הותר לו אלא כדי צורכו וחיותו ואם די לו בשתיה לא יאכל ואם די לו
באכילה פעם אחת לא יאכל שתי פעמים, ולא יותר ממה שצריך" עכ"ל. וכן
הכף החיים בסי' תקנ"ו אות ט' בענין הבדלה של חולה בט' באב שחל ביום
ראשון פסק דאם אינו צריך לאכול בלילה ימתין עד הבוקר ואז יבדיל.

ולכאורה קשה על כל הפוסקים הנ"ל, הרי חז"ל לא גזרו כלל על חולה ואם
כן מדוע החולה מוגבל בכמות או בזמן האכילה הרי אינו מצווה להתענות
כלל?

ושמעתי מהגר"ד ליאור שאפשר לומר שאמנם חז"ל לא גזרו על החולה
להתענות כלל בט"ב אבל הוא אינו בגדר של חולה שמותר לו לאכול עד
שהוא צריך לאכול. לדוגמא: אם החולה או היולדת אינם צריכים לאכול עד
השעה עשר בבקר, אם כן עד שעה זו אין להם היתר לאכול כי עדיין אינם
בגדר חולה שצריך לאכול. רק מאותה השעה הם בגדר חולה שחז"ל לא
גזרו עליו. ובזה אפשר להבין שעל אף שחז"ל לא גזרו על החולה להתענות
מ"מ הפוסקים כתבו שעד שהוא צריך לאכול יש לו להתענות.

37. מגן אברהם סי' תקנ"ד ס"ק ט'.

פרק 18

1. שו"ע או"ח סי' רי"ט סע' א' ומ"ב שם ס"ק ב' והולך כבר על בוריו". וכתב
הכף החיים סי' רי"ט אות ז': ולפ"ז יולדת אינה מברכת הגומל עד לאחר ז'
כי אז נתרפאת לגמרי והרי היא כשאר כל אדם כמ"ש לקמן סי' תרי"ז
סי' ד' יעו"ש" עכ"ל.

2. מ"ב שם ס"ק ח', וראה תורת היולדת פרק ס"ב סע' ה' שהביא דעה שדוקא
אחר ל' יום יש לברך וע"ש. וראה בספר תודת חיים מהרב נסים ששון
עמ' ע"ח שכתב שאם מרגשת בעצמה שהיא עדיין חלושה נכון להמתין עד
שתרגיש בריאה לגמרי.

3. עיין כף החיים שם אות ג'. ועיין שו"ת יחוה דעת ח"ד סי' ט"ו. ועיין קצות
השולחן ח"ב סי' ב'.

4. שו"ת חתם סופר או"ח סי' נ"א ובכף החיים אות י"ד ובן איש חי ש"א פרק
עקב אות ג' והטעם הוא, כי הברכה נתקנה במקום זבח תודה, ותודה אינה
אלא ביום. טעם נוסף הוא מפני שבברכה זו נקראת הלל, והלל אינו אלא
ביום. וכן כתב החת"ס הנ"ל בשם אליהו רבה.

5. שו"ת ציץ אליעזר חי"ג סי' י"ז. ועיין שם שכתב דבגברים אין להתיר לברך
לכתחלה בלילה ובדיעבד אם בירך בלילה בודאי שיצא. ובנשים יש להתיר
לכתחלה לברך בלילה.

6. בן איש חי ש"א פרק עקב אות ג' וז"ל "והמברך עומד משום דברכה זו היא
במקום קרבן תודה והמקריב עומד ומקריב". וגם מפני שהוא כהלל כמ"ש
החת"ס בשם א"ר וכן פסק המ"ב בס"ק ד'.

7. עיין בן איש חי שם אות ה' וז"ל "ואם קשה לה לברך בעשרה מחמת
הבושה תברך בלא שם ומלכות", עכ"ל. ובמ"ב שם ס"ק ג' כתב "וגם הנשים
מנהג העולם שאין מברכין ברכה זו וכתבו האחרונים הטעם משום דסדר
ברכה זו הוא בפני עשרה ולאו אורח ארעא לאשה. ויש שכתבו דמ"מ נכון
הוא שתתברך בפני עשרה עכ"פ בפני נשים ואיש אחד", עכ"ל. ובס"ק י"ז
הביא עצה אחרת שהבעל יברך בנוכחותה "הגומל לחייבים טובות שגמלך
כל טוב" וכשהיא תענה אמן יוצאת בזה, ואם בירך שלא בפניה יאמר
"שגמל לאשתי כל טוב". אולם כף החיים אות כ"ז חולק עליו וז"ל "וכתב
הב"י הא דאחר מברך דוקא על רפואת רבו אבל למי שאינו רבו אעפ"י
שהוא חביב עליו כגון כגון אשתו שילדה וכדומה אינו מברך על רפואתו
ואם בירך גורעין בו דדילמא ברכה לבטלה היא", עכ"ל. והנה הדרכי משר

באות א' כתב בשם הריא"ז דאם אדם רוצה לברך הגומל על אוהבו ועל קרובו שהוא כואב עליו הרשות בידו. וכן פסק בהגה סע' ד'. וכן פסק הב"ח דיש רשות לכתחלה לברך על אוהביו או קרובו כמו באביו ורבו וכל שכן אשתו ובניו, כי אין תועלת לאדם יותר מהצלת אשתו שהיא כגופו והוא הדין הצלת בניו ואוהביו, ולדעת הב"ח זוהי ג"כ דעתו של הרשב"א. אך באליהו רבה באות י"א חלק עליו בזה וסובר שלדעת הרשב"א אפשר לברך רק על אביו או רבו. ובאות י"ב כתב "שטעם מנהג הנשים שלא לברך כדאיתא בזוהר פ' אמור ובש"ס בכמה דוכתא דעיקר עונש אשה בחטא בעלה כמו קטן. [אולם אפשר לחלק ולומר שדוקא בשאר סכנות אבל בלידה המשנה בשבת (פ"ב ו') אומרת "על שלש עבירות נשים מתות בשעת לידתן: על שאינן זהירות בנדה חלה ובהדלקת הנר", ע"כ עונש אשה בשעת לידה הוא מחמת עצמה וא"כ שפיר מברכת.] לכן נ"ל דיותר טוב דבעל יאמר 'אשר גמלך כל טוב' והיא תענה אמן. ואף שהעליתי לעיל דאוהביו וקרוביו לא יברכו מ"מ בזה יש לסמוך על הפוסקים דמברכין דאשתו דאשתו כגופו וע"ל ס"ק ה' [שם הבא עצה אחרת דכשהבעל עולה לתורה ואומר ברכו יכוין שנותן הודאה בשביל אשתו והיא תענה אמן על ברכתו.] ועיין בכף החיים אות כ"ח ומ"א ס"ק ג' דגם על אביו ורבו אין נוהגים עכשיו לברך, והטעם הוא משום שזה פגם בכבוד אביו ורבו לומר 'החייבים'. ולכאורה טעם זה אינו שייך באשתו, וא"כ שפיר מברך בשבילה. וכן כתב הערוך השולחן בסע' ט' דיכול הבעל לברך שגמלך כל טוב והיא תענה אמן דאין לך אהבה ונוגע בטובתה יותר ממנו דאשתו דאשתו כגופו, דלא כיש מי שמפקפק בזה ומ"מ אין המנהג כן", עכ"ל. לפיכך לעדות המזרח בודאי שאין לבעל לברך על אשתו. ולאשכנזים הדבר נתון למורי הוראה. ולדעתו של הגר"מ אליהו גם לאשכנזים אין לברך על אשתו בשם ומלכות.

פרק 19

פרק 20

16. מפי ד"ר מתתיהו ארליכמן. רא' שו"ת ציץ אליעזר חי"ג פ"ב שכתב בשם
ד"ר אברהם שחום של 37.5 מע' צליוס ואפילו פחות מזה נחשב לחום גבוה
לענין זה.

17. שו"ת אג"מ יו"ד ח"ב סי' קכ"א. וראה שו"ת צ"א חי"ג פ"ב.

18. שו"ע יו"ד סי' רס"ג, סע' א'.

19. שמעתי מהרב יוסף דוד ויסברג בשם הרב י.ש. אלישיב והרב שלמה זלמן
אויערבך.

20. כי הוא נחשב חולה.

21. שו"ת ציץ אליעזר חי"ג סי' פ"א.

22. שו"ת אג"מ יו"ד ח"ב סי' קכ"א.

23. בראשית י"ז, ט'.

24. ספר החינוך מצוה ב'.

25. בראשית י"ז, י"ב.

26. שבת ק"ל, א'.

פרק 21

1. ספר מטעמים, מערכת יולדת ועיין בדגול מרבבה יו"ד ס"ס קע"ח שכתב
"לפירוש התרומת הדשן שהביא רמ"א לקמן סי' רס"ה סע' י"ב דהיינו בליל
שבת ולפי ששכיחי בבתים ע' תה"ד סי' רס"ט קשה למה אין עושין סעודה גם
לנקבה שגם כן נמלטה מרחם," עכ"ל. ובספר מרגליות הים סנהדרין ל"ב ב'
על "שבוע הבן שבוע הבן" כתב וז"ל יעיין בהלכות רבינו יצחק אבן גאות
(שערי שמחה ח"ב ע' ל"ח) שכתב: ובאבל תניא יתומה לשאת וכו' שבוע הבת
ושבוע הבן קודם כו', וכן הביא הרמב"ן בתורת האדם [ווינציאה שנ"ה ל"ג
סע"ג] ממכילתא אחריתא דאבל שבוע הבת ושבוע הבן וכו', וראה
בתוספתא עתיקתא ח"ב ע' מ"ד, נראה כי כל השבוע משנולד בן או בת חגגו
כל ערב בהדלקת נרות ושמחה. ויתכן שגם בגמרא לפנינו צ"ל שבוע הבן
שבוע הבת [ולא נקטו שבוע הבן בכפילא ללא צורך] וכן אור הנר ברבור
חיל משתה שם - לבן - משתה שם - לבת" עכ"ל. לכאורה לפי זה יש לעשות
את השמחה בתוך השבוע הראשון, אבל העולם לא נהגו כך.

2. עבודה זרה כ"ז, א'.

3. ספר החינוך מצוה ב'.

4. שמות י"ט, ג'.

5. מדרש רבה שם.

6. מהר"ל דרוש על התורה (מהדורת ירושלים עמ' כ"ז).

7. משלי ל"א, כ"ז וראה פירוש הגר"א.

8. משלי שם, כ"ו.

9. סנהדרין ק', ב'.

10. שם.

11. במדבר רבה י"א, ה'.

12. בבא מציעא נ"ט, א'.

פרק 22

1. ושם רשעים ירקב, יומא ל"ח, ב' וראה ספר אוצר הברית לרב יוסף דוד ויסברג בקונטרס זה שמי לעולם פרק ה' סע' א.

2. דרכי תשובה סי' קע"ח ס"ק י"ד וז"ל "עיין בשו"ת מהר"ם שיק שם סי' קס"ט שהרעיש על מה שיש בני אדם שמכנים עצמם בשם הגוים כי בודאי יש בזה איסור דאורייתא מקרא ד'ואבדיל אתכם מן העמים להיות לי' דאין רשאי לדמות להם בשום ענין וכמו שאסור לדמות להם במלבושם ובהליכותם ובשאר מנהגיהם מכ"ש דאסור לדמות בשמם עיי"ש באריכות".

3. שו"ת צפנת פענח סי' רע"ה הובא בספר אוצר הברית בקונטרס זה שמי לעולם סי' ו', סע' א.

4. שו"ת עין יהודה סי' י"ב, הובא בספר אוצר הברית בקונטרס זה שמי לעולם, פרק ד', א', ועיין עוד בתורה תמימה בראשית ל"ב אות ד' וז"ל דמפני שאנו נעים ונדים בגלות ראוי לנו לזכור השתלשלות יחוסי אבות על ידי שהאבות יקראו לבניהם בשם אבותיהם המנוחים וכמו שנוהגים בזה"ז. וגם בתלמוד מצינו מנהג זה בכ"מ, עכ"ל.

5. ועיין אוצר הברית שם דף ר"ח - ר"כ.

6. ועיין בשו"ת אגרות משה יו"ד ח"ב סי' קכ"ב.

7. ועיין מגיד מישרים פרשת שמות, ועיין שם בענין שם דיהושע (עמ' 106, מהדורת יחיאל אברהם בר לב.)

8. רות רבה ב', ה': "מחלון שנמחו מן העולם וכליון שכלו מן העולם".

9. ועיין רש"י בראשית כ"ה, כ"ו ד"ה "ויקרא שמו יעקב" שגם יעקב נקרא שמו ע"י הקב"ה.

10. עמוד שמים עמ' ד' אות כ"ג מובא בקונטרס "זה שמי לעולם".

11. עיין בשו"ת ציץ אליעזר ח"ג סי' כ', שפסק שיש לקרוא השם בקריאת התורה הראשונה. ועיין בשו"ת מנחת יצחק חי"ג סי' כ' שהביא שלשה מנהגים בזה.

פרק 23

19. שו"ע יו"ד סי' פ"א סע' ז' ברמ"א ועיין שם בט"ז וש"ך. ועיין בדרכי תשובה שם ס"ק צ' שהביא מהשדי חמד דאף שיונק ממינקת ישראלית צריך להשתדל שתהא המינקת בעלת מדות טובות, לא רעשנית ולא רגזנית. ובס"ק צ"א כתב וז"ל "ולפ"ז בתינוק שרוצה לינק דבודאי אין בו שום הבנה יש להקל בכ"מ ובכל גווני אבל פשוט הוא דכ"ז הוא מדינא אבל מחשש שמטמטם הלב יש לזה אף בקטן שאינו בר הבנה כלל וכו'" ע"ש.

20. ברכות כ'.

21. ויקרא רבה י"ד.

22. גיטין פ"א, א.

23. שו"ע או"ח סי' ע"ה מ"ב ס"ק ג'.

24. שם מ"ב ס"ק ה', ועיין שם ס"ק ד'.

25. שו"ע או"ח סי' ע"ד סע' ד', וסי' ע"ה סע' א' ברמ"א.

26. שמירת שבת כהלכתה פרק א', סע' נ'.

27. כתובות ל"ט, א'.

28. שו"ע סי' שכ"ח סע' ל"ד ואסור משום מפרק.

29. שו"ע או"ח סי' ש"ל סע' ח' ומ"ב שם ס"ק ל"ב דאין זה כדרך מפרק כיון
שהולך לאיבוד, ועוד דהוי מלאכה שאינה צריכה לגופה דפטור ומשום
צערא לא גזרינן כמו מפיס מורסא. וראה שמירת שבת כהלכתה פרק ל"ו
סע' כ', ובספר אוצר דינים לאשה ולבת סי' י"ז סע' כ"ב.

30. שמירת שבת כהלכתה פרק ל"ו סע' כ' ועיין שם בהערה שיש להקפיד שלא
יצטבר לשיעור של גרוגרת שהוא כשליש ביצה שהוא 19.2 סמ"ק (לפי הגר"ח
נאה) או 33.3 סמ"ק (לפי החזו"א). ובשם הגרש"ז אויערבך כתב שצריך
לרוקן את המשאבה למקום שהחלב הולך לאיבוד דאל"כ יצטרף לשיעור.

31. שו"ע או"ח סי' שכ"ח סע' ל"ה ועיין בשעה"צ שם.

32. שמירת שבת כהלכתה פרק ל"ו סע' כ"א, ועיין חזון איש או"ח סי' נ"ט
אות ג' ושו"ת הר צבי או"ח סי' כ"א דדוקא פחות פחות מכפית וחצי שזהו
פחות מכשיעור.

33. שו"ע או"ח סי' שכ"ח סע' כ"ב.

34. שמירת שבת כהלכתה פרק ל"ט סע' י"ז על פי כה"ח סי' תרי"ז אות ב'.

פרק 24

1. באר היטב או"ח סי' רס"ב ס"ק ב'. וכתב שהסיבה לכך נמצאת בכתבי האר"י ז"ל.
2. סידור בית יעקב (לר' יעקב עמדין) מנהגי ליל שבת.
3. נדה ל"א א'.
4. סידור בית יעקב מנהגי ליל שבת.
5. אוצר דינים ומנהגים, ברכת הבנים עמ' 56 בשם פחד יצחק.
6. בראשית מ"ח, כ'.
7. מועד קטן כ"ח, א'.

פרק 26

1. שבת ל"א, א'.
2. ביצה ט"ז, א'.
3. דברים י"א, י"ט.
4. קידושין ל' א', רמב"ם הל' תלמוד תורה פ"א הל' ב' ו"ג, שו"ע יו"ד סי' רמ"ה
סע' א'.
5. דברים ו', ז'.
6. ברכות י"ז, א'.
7. מכילתא פרשת יתרו כ', כ'.
8. שמות כ"ה, כ'.
9. במדבר רבה י"ב.
10. וכן כתוב "ויגרש את האדם וישכן מקדם לגן עדן את הכרובים ואת להט
החרב המתהפכת לשמור את דרך עץ החיים" (בראשית ג' כ"ד) "ואין עץ
חיים אלא תורה" - ברכות ל"ב, ב'.
11. בראשית ב', י"א וי"ב.
12. בראשית רבה ט"ז, ד'.
13. ישעיהו ב', ג'.

Glossary

The following glossary provides a partial explanation of some of the Hebrew and Aramaic (A.) words and phrases used in this book. The spellings and explanations reflect the way the specific word is used herein. Often, there are alternate spellings and meanings for the words.

AM YISRAEL: the People of Israel.

BEDIKAH: an examination for ritual purity.

BERACHAH: a blessing.

BEIS HAMIKDASH: the Holy Temple.

BIRKAS HA-GOMEL: the blessing recited after surviving a dangerous experience.

BIRKAS HA-MAZON: the Grace after Meals.

BNEI YISRAEL: the Children of Israel.

CHAZAL: the Hebrew acronym for "our Sages of blessed memory."

CHOK: a statute of the Torah.

D'RABBANAN: (A.) according to the Rabbis.

D'ORAYSA: (A.) according to the Torah.

DERASH: interpretation; exposition.

HAKADOSH BARUCH HU: the Holy One, blessed be He.

HA-MOTZI LECHEM MIN HA-ARETZ: "Who brings forth bread from the earth," the blessing recited over bread.

HAVDALAH: the blessing recited at the conclusion of Sabbaths and Festivals.

KIDDUSH: sanctification of the Sabbath and Festivals, usually recited over a cup of wine.

KIDDUSH HASHEM: sanctification of the Divine Name.

LECHEM MISHNEH: the two loaves of bread placed on the Sabbath table.

MASHIACH: the Messiah.

MIDDOS: good attributes.

MIKVEH: a ritual bath.

MOTZAEI SHABBOS: the end of the Sabbath; Saturday night.

MUKTZEH: [an object that is] set aside as unusable on Shabbos.

NESHAMAH: the soul.

NETILAS YADAYIM: the ritual of washing the hands.

NIDDAH: the condition of menstrual impurity.

OLAM HA-BA: the World to Come.

P'RU U'REVU: "Be fruitful and multiply" (Bereshis 1:28).

PIDYON HA-BEN: the ceremony of the redemption of the firstborn son.

PIKUACH NEFESH: a matter of life and death.

POSEK (POSKIM): halachic authority (-ties).

RASHA: an evil person.

SHECHINAH: the Divine Presence.

SHINUI: lit., a change; performing an act in a manner different from the way it is usually done.

SHIRAH: song, poetry.

SHIURIM: lit., amount or measure; the maximum amounts halachically permissible for a sick person to eat or drink on a fast day.

SHOMER SHABBOS: Sabbath-observant.

SIMCHAH: happiness; a joyous occasion.

TAHARAH: ritual purity.

TALMID CHACHAM: a Torah scholar; a learned man.

TEMEH MES: the condition of ritual impurity after coming in contact with the dead.

TECHIYAS HA-MESIM: the resurrection of the dead.

TEHILLIM: (the Book of) Psalms.

TESHUVAH: repentance.

TUMAH: ritual impurity.

VESES: menstruation.

YETZER HA-RA: the evil inclination.

YOLEDES: a woman who has just given birth.

YOM TOV: a Jewish Festival.

Glossary of Medical Terms

ABORTION (MISCARRIAGE): the interruption of pregnancy with the expulsion of the fetus before the twentieth week of pregnancy.

ABRUPTIO PLACENTAE: the partial or complete separation of the placenta from the uterine wall.

ALPHA FETOPROTEIN (AFP): a protein produced by the fetal liver which passes into the mother's blood via the placenta.

AMNIOTIC FLUID: the liquid contained in the amniotic sac in which the fetus lies during gestation. The fluid serves to protect the fetus from injury and maintain even temperature.

AMNIOTOMY: the artificial rupture of the amniotic sac.

ANEMIA: a condition in which there is a reduction of the number of red blood cells, or of the total amount of hemoglobin in the bloodstream, or of both.

ANTIBODY: a protein produced in the immune system which responds to and defends against an antigen (foreign substance) in the body.

ANTI-D (RHESUS GAMMAGLOBULIN): a serum which prevents an Rh-negative mother from producing antibodies that would attack and destroy blood cells in an Rh-positive fetus.

BILIRUBIN: a yellowish pigment formed by the destruction of red blood cells. Although the bilirubin is normally excreted through the bowel, if the amount of bilirubin is excessive a yellowish tinge to the skin may result.

BRAXTON HICKS CONTRACTIONS: "false" uterine contractions which are mild and irregular, occurring intermittently during the third trimester of pregnancy.

BREECH PRESENTATION: the presentation of the buttocks or feet first in childbirth.

CERVICAL DILATION: the gradual widening of the neck of the uterus.

CHROMOSOMES: rod-shaped structures in the nucleus of a cell which carry hereditary factors.

CROWNING: the appearance of the baby's head at the vaginal opening prior to delivery.

DEHYDRATION: the excessive loss of body fluids.

DIABETES (MELLITUS): a disorder characterized by an overabundance of blood sugar due to insufficient insulin production in the pancreas or inability of the body to utilize insulin.

DIZYGOTIC: fraternal twins who are the product of two ova and two sperm.

ECTOPIC PREGNANCY: a condition in which the fertilized egg implants itself outside the uterus, usually in the fallopian tubes.

EDEMA: a localized or generalized condition in which body tissues contain an excessive amount of fluid, most commonly manifested in lower-leg swelling.

EFFACEMENT: the thinning out of the cervix which precedes or coincides with cervical dilation.

EMBRYO: the prenatal stage of the developing human from fertilization through eight weeks.

ENGAGEMENT: when the fetal head descends to the level of the ischial spines in the pelvis.

ENGORGEMENT: the build-up of fluid in the lymphatic and venous circulation, causing breasts to be full, heavy and hard.

EPISIOTOMY: an incision made during the second stage of delivery to widen the vaginal orifice.

ESTROGEN: a hormone produced by the ovary, adrenal glands and placenta. Estrogen is responsible for the development of secondary sex characteristics, menstruation and pregnancy.

FETUS: an unborn baby from eight weeks of pregnancy.

HEMOGLOBIN: the iron-containing pigment of red blood cells which carry oxygen from the lungs to the tissues. The amount of hemoglobin for adult females averages 12-16 gr./100 ml. of blood; adult males, 14-18 gr./100 ml. of blood.

HYPERTENSION: high blood pressure.

INSULIN: a hormone secreted by the beta cells of the pancreas which is responsible for the proper metabolism of blood sugar (glucose).

JAUNDICE: a condition characterized by a yellow discoloration of skin and eyes due to excess bilirubin in the blood.

LIGHTENING: the engagement of the fetal head, usually occurring in primiparas about two weeks before delivery.

MECONIUM: the greenish-black waste product which accumulates in the fetus' intestines and is excreted shortly after birth.

MONOZYGOTIC: identical twins from an ovum which divided after fertilization.

MOULDING: the shaping of the fetal head as it adapts itself to the pelvis and birth canal.

MULTIPARA: a woman who has given birth more than one time.

OSTEOPOROSIS: the increased porosity and softening of the bones associated with aging.

OVULATION: the release of the ovum about fourteen days before menstruation.

OVUM: an egg cell released monthly from the ovary.

OXYTOCIN: a pituitary hormone that stimulates the uterus to contract and acts on the mammary gland to stimulate the release of milk.

PAP SMEAR (PAPANICOLAOU SMEAR): the microscopic examination of cells shed from the cervix.

PLACENTA PREVIA: a condition in which the placenta implants at the lower segment of the uterus, partially or fully covering the cervical opening. Can cause hemorrhage during the third trimester and often necessitates delivery of the baby by cesarean section.

PRIMIPARA: a woman giving birth for the first time.

PROGESTERONE: a hormone which is responsible for changes in the uterine lining to prepare it for implantation of the fertilized ovum.

PROSTAGLANDINS: fatty acid derivatives which are hormone-like, secreted by many body tissues. They affect smooth muscle, which causes the uterus to contract.

QUICKENING: when fetal movements are felt for the first time, at approximately the eighteenth to twenty-second week of pregnancy.

RESPIRATORY DISTRESS SYNDROME (RDS): formerly known as hyaline membrane disease. Lung impairment where ventilation and medical support are necessary to maintain breathing. Common in premature infants.

RH FACTOR: a group of antigens present in the red blood cells of those who have an Rh-positive blood type, which are capable of destroying red blood cells in those whose blood is Rh-negative.

TAY-SACHS DISEASE: a hereditary disease that progressively destroys cells of the central nervous system, caused by a congenital enzyme deficiency. It is an autosomal recessive disorder (inherited from two carrier parents) which is fatal by the age of five years.

TERATOGEN: any substance or environmental agent that can damage the developing fetus.

Hebrew Childbirth Lexicon

English	Transliteration	Hebrew
abdomen	*beten*	בֶּטֶן
amniotic fluid	*mei shafir*	מֵי שָׁפִיר
anesthesia	*hardamah*	הַרְדָּמָה
bladder	*shalpuchit ha-sheten*	שַׁלְפּוּחִית הַשֶּׁתֶן
blood pressure	*lachatz dam*	לַחַץ־דָּם
breasts	*shadayim*	שָׁדַיִם
cervix	*tzavar ha-rechem*	צַוָּאר הָרֶחֶם
check-up	*bedikah*	בְּדִיקָה
contractions	*tzirim*	צִירִים
cramp(s)	*hitkavtzut (-tzuyot)*	הִתְכַּוְּצוּת (-צֻיּוֹת)
dilation	*petichah*	פְּתִיחָה
effacement	*mechikah*	מְחִיקָה
enema	*choken*	חֹקֶן
fallopian tube(s)	*chatzotzrah (-rot)*	חֲצוֹצְרָה (-רוֹת)
fertilization	*hafrayah*	הַפְרָיָה
fetal development	*hitpatchut ha-ubar*	הִתְפַּתְּחוּת הָעֻבָּר
gynecologist	*rofeh nashim*	רוֹפֵא נָשִׁים
heartbeat	*pe'imat ha-lev*	פְּעִימַת הַלֵּב
infection	*daleket*	דַּלֶּקֶת
injection	*zerikah*	זְרִיקָה
intravenous transfusion (I.V.)	*erui*	עֵרוּי
jaundice	*tzahevet*	צַהֶבֶת
nipples	*pitmot*	פִּטְמוֹת
operation (cesarean)	*nituach (keisari)*	נִתּוּחַ (קֵיסָרִי)
ovaries	*shachalot*	שַׁחֲלוֹת
pain(s)	*ke'ev (im)*	כְּאֵב (ים)

pregnancy	herayon	הֵרָיוֹן
pressure	lachatz	לַחַץ
pulse	dofek	דֹּפֶק
push (n.)	lechitzah	לְחִיצָה
pediatrician	rofeh yeladim	רוֹפֵא יְלָדִים
rupture of membranes	pekiat mei shafir	פְּקִיעַת מֵי שָׁפִיר
shave	giluach	גִּלּוּחַ
umbilical cord	chevel ha-tabur	חֶבֶל הַטַּבּוּר
ultrasound test	bedikah al-kolit	בְּדִיקָה עַל-קוֹלִית
uterus	rechem	רֶחֶם
vaccination	chisun	חִסּוּן
weight	mishkal	מִשְׁקָל
x-ray	tzilum	צִלּוּם

Index

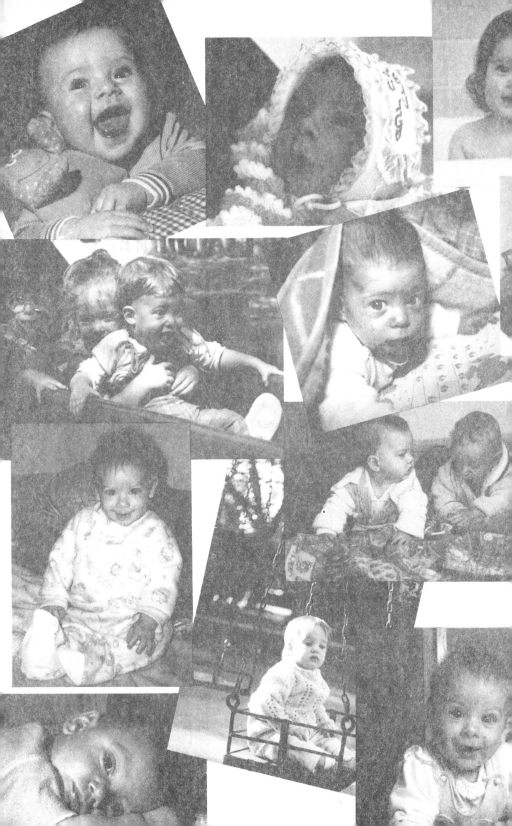